the**facts**

obsessive–
compulsive
disorder

also available in the**facts** series

the**facts**

obsessive–compulsive disorder

FOURTH EDITION

STANLEY J. RACHMAN

Psychology Department, University of
British Columbia, Vancouver

and

†PADMAL DE SILVA

Institute of Psychiatry, King's College,
University of London
South London and Maudsley National Health
Service Trust, London

OXFORD
UNIVERSITY PRESS

OXFORD
UNIVERSITY PRESS

Great Clarendon Street, Oxford OX2 6DP

Oxford University Press is a department of the University of Oxford.
It furthers the University's objective of excellence in research, scholarship,
and education by publishing worldwide in

Oxford New York

Auckland Cape Town Dar es Salaam Hong Kong Karachi
Kuala Lumpur Madrid Melbourne Mexico City Nairobi
New Delhi Shanghai Taipei Toronto

With offices in

Argentina Austria Brazil Chile Czech Republic France Greece
Guatemala Hungary Italy Japan Poland Portugal Singapore
South Korea Switzerland Thailand Turkey Ukraine Vietnam

Oxford is a registered trade mark of Oxford University Press
in the UK and in certain other countries

Published in the United States
by Oxford University Press Inc., New York

© Oxford University Press 2009

The moral rights of the authors have been asserted
Database right Oxford University Press (maker)

First edition published 1992
Second edition published 1998
Third edition published 2004
Fourth edition published 2009

British Library Cataloguing in Publication Data

Data available

Library of Congress Cataloguing in Publication Data

Data available

Typeset in Plantin
by Cepha Imaging Pvt. Ltd., Bangalore, India
Printed in Great Britain by
Ashford Colour Press Ltd, Gosport, Hampshire

ISBN 978–0–19–956177–3

10 9 8 7 6 5 4 3 2 1

Whilst every effort has been made to ensure that the contents of this book are as complete, accurate,
and up-to-date as possible at the date of writing, Oxford University Press is not able to give any
guarantee or assurance that such is the case. Readers are urged to take appropriately qualified
medical advice in all cases. The information in this book is intended to be useful to the general
reader, but should not be used as a means of self-diagnosis or for the prescription of medication.

Foreword

Exactly 7 years ago, in January 2002, I was diagnosed with an illness that left me bewildered, confused and feeling as if I was the only person in the world that was suffering from it: this illness was obsessive–compulsive disorder.

Over the following months I read many books about obsessive–compulsive disorder, and I searched for an understanding that I was unable to find elsewhere. It was only when I was recommended an earlier version of this publication did I discover a book that truly allowed me to understand obsessive–compulsive disorder.

So when I was offered the opportunity and privilege of writing a foreword for this new edition of *Obsessive–Compulsive Disorder: The Facts* I jumped at the chance. I believe that this book will lead others affected by OCD to a better understanding of what they're dealing with and to a much greater chance of recovery.

Over the years there have been many books written on the subject of this still frequently misunderstood, debilitating illness, yet none have remained so balanced and unbiased or managed to pack so much evidence-based content in such a structured way as this book does. This latest edition is no exception and continues to build on its predecessors by offering even clearer laid out content.

One of OCD-UK's key objectives is to empower sufferers to make positive steps towards recovery and *Obsessive–Compulsive Disorder: The Facts* continues to be a vital tool in helping our charity towards that goal.

Obsessive–Compulsive Disorder: The Facts offers the reader a clear and concise guide to understanding obsessive–compulsive disorder by simply presenting the facts.

Perhaps the essential compliment I can pay this book is that it is truly the definitive guide to understanding obsessive–compulsive disorder. It will always be the first book on my suggested list of reading material for health professionals, sufferers, and carers alike.

Ashley Fulwood
Chief-Executive of OCD-UK
www.ocduk.org
January 2009

Preface

This book is intended to provide the reader with basic information about obsessive–compulsive disorders. The main features of this anxiety disorder are *obsessions*—recurrent, unwanted, unwelcome, upsetting intrusive thoughts that are unacceptable and even repugnant—and *compulsive behaviour*, those repetitive, purposeful actions that the person feels compelled to carry out (such as compulsive washing), even though he recognizes that they are irrational and/ or excessive. The disorder usually arises in early adulthood and is often associated with depression. It is estimated that the chances of a person developing an obsessive–compulsive disorder at some point in his lifetime are in the region of 1–2%. It is customary to rank the seriousness of the disorder from *mild*–unpleasant and annoying but manageable—to *severe* cases, which are distressing and dominate the person's life. People who have a mild disorder can cope with it reasonably well, and generally need relatively minimal professional help. Those who are severely affected invariably need a considerable amount of professional help, often over a lengthy period. People who have a moderate form of the disorder usually improve significantly when they receive the appropriate psychological treatment.

We have been involved in the study and treatment of obsessive–compulsive patients for many years. In our clinical practice, we find it essential to provide a good deal of information about this often puzzling disorder to sufferers and their families, and hence decided to write this book. The First Edition was published in 1992, and happily in the past few years there have been important advances in knowledge and the provision of professional help that need to be brought to the attention of readers. This Fourth Edition is an expanded version in which we have added essential, up-to-date information.

In recognition of the important advances that have been made in the treatment of depression and anxiety disorders, of which obsessive–compulsive disorder is one, in October 2007 the Minister of Health announced a massive expansion in the provision of psychological treatment facilities in the UK.

'Psychological therapies have proved to be as effective as drugs in tackling these common mental health problems and are often more effective in the long run.' The target is to train an additional 8000 psychological therapists in the near future. The aim is to reduce the average waiting time from the current 18 months to a few weeks as the service rolls out. The training of new therapists is under way, and information about the availability of services can be obtained from NHS websites and other sources. It is preferable to consult your family practiner first, but self-referrals are now acceptable.

Research in the last 30 years has added a great amount to our knowledge about obsessive–compulsive disorder, and we have attempted to give a summary of the major findings. Much of what is said about the treatment of obsessive–compulsive disorder in these pages reflects a psychological orientation. This is partly because of our professional training but, more importantly, because the psychological approach has provided the most effective treatment strategies to help people who have these problems. Current and future research will no doubt lead to the refinement of the existing therapeutic strategies and the development of new ones. It will also throw more light on the causes of obsessive–compulsive disorders, and related questions. Like everyone else in this field, we eagerly await these developments.

Note

Because of the problem of gender in the English language, we have had to decide whether to use 'he', 'she', or 'person' when referring to people. Different authors have different practices, and we are aware that some people have strong views on this issue. For ease of reading, we have retained the more conventional, male form.

London and   P. de S.
Vancouver   S. R.
2008.

Acknowledgements

We wish to thank Professor Rosamund Shafran, Dr Adam Radomsky, Dr Clare Philips, and Dr Maureen Whittal for their valuable assistance. In addition we thank Dona de Silva for her excellent secretarial help, and express our gratitude to the staff of Oxford University Press for their unvarying support and advice. We are indebted to many colleagues and students, past and present, who have contributed to our thinking on this disorder.

Contents

1

Obsessive–compulsive disorder: what is it?

> ## ➲ Key points
>
> ♦ Obsessive–compulsive disorders are psychological disorders.
>
> ♦ The most common features are obsessions and compulsive behaviour.
>
> ♦ Obsessions are defined and described.
>
> ♦ Compulsive behaviour is defined and described.
>
> ♦ A diagnosis of obsessive–compulsive disorder is made on the basis of the person's complaints, detailed interviews, and psychological tests.
>
> ♦ It is customary to classify the disorders into mild, moderate, and severe cases.
>
> ♦ In severe cases the patient experiences considerable distress and disability.
>
> ♦ Obsessive–compulsive disorders develop in late adolescence or early adulthood.
>
> ♦ Approximately 1.6% of the population develop the disorder.

Obsessive–compulsive disorder has been traditionally regarded as a neurotic disorder, like phobias and anxiety states. Other terms used for this disorder include: 'obsessive (or obsessional)–compulsive neurosis' and 'obsessive (or obsessional)–compulsive illness'—or simply 'obsessive (or obsessional) disorder' or 'compulsive disorder'. It can interfere with one's life, and people with this problem suffer considerable distress, and often feel that they are helpless and hopeless. They are afflicted with disturbing unwanted thoughts and feel compelled repeatedly to carry out activities that they know to be irrational. It is difficult for them to understand, and equally difficult to explain to other people, why they repeatedly engage in senseless behaviour. The fact that their obsessive–compulsive problems are so puzzling as to defy explanation is an added burden, and can erode one's self-esteem. Neurotic disorders are generally considered to be less handicapping and disabling than psychotic illnesses—such as schizophrenia—but severe obsessive–compulsive disorder can cause great distress and major incapacitation.

Patients who suffer from anxiety disorders, such as obsessive–compulsive disorder, are aware that they have a psychological problem that leads them to think and behave irrationally in particular circumstances. In all other respects their intellectual abilities and ability to reason are unimpaired. Most sufferers are able to function at least moderately well: they are able to work, maintain family and other relationships, and pursue their goals and interests. In contrast, most people afflicted with major mental illnesses, psychotic disorders, such as schizophrenia, suffer from numerous and chronic impairments. Many of them have limited insight into what is wrong, and their contact with the outside world may be seriously distorted. Their relationships with other people tend to be unsatisfying and unsatisfactory.

The terms 'neurotic disorders' and 'neuroses' are not widely used any more, and have been replaced by the term 'anxiety disorders'. Obsessive–compulsive disorder is now classified as one of these anxiety disorders. Other disorders that are included are: phobias, panic disorder, post-traumatic stress disorders, social phobias, agoraphobia, and generalized anxiety stress disorder. Intense and poorly controlled anxiety is the basic feature of these disorders, and there is overlap of symptoms among them. The types of anxiety disorder are set out in Table 1.1.

Table 1.1 Anxiety disorders

Panic disorder, with or without agoraphobia
Agoraphobia, without a history of panics
Social phobia
Specific phobia
Generalized anxiety disorder
Obsessive–compulsive disorder
Post-traumatic stress disorder
Acute stress disorder

Table 1.2 Summary of criteria widely used for the diagnosis of obsessive–compulsive disorder

---

1. The person must have either obsessions or compulsions or both.

   (a) *Obsessions* are recurrent, persistent ideas, thoughts, images, or impulses that intrude into consciousness and are experienced as senseless or repugnant. They form against one's will, and the person usually attempts to resist them, or get rid of them. The person recognizes that they are his own thoughts. They also cause marked anxiety or distress.

   (b) *Compulsions* are repetitive, purposeful forms of behaviour that are carried out because of a strong feeling of compulsion to do so. The goal is to prevent or reduce anxiety or distress, or to prevent some dreaded event or situation. However, the activity is not connected in a realistic way with what it is aimed to prevent, or it is clearly excessive. The person generally recognizes the senselessness of the behaviour and does not get pleasure from carrying out the activity, although it provides a relief from tension. Compulsions are usually performed according to certain rules or in a stereotyped fashion.

---

2. They are not due to another disorder, such as schizophrenia, depression or organic mental disorder.

---

3. The obsessions and/or compulsions cause distress to the person and/or interfere with his life and activities.

What is meant when someone is described as having an obsessive–compulsive disorder? The person displays and/or complains of either obsessions or compulsions or both, to a degree that affects his everyday functioning or causes him distress. Diagnosis of the condition is made on this basis (Table 1.2).

What are obsessions?

An obsession is a recurrent, unwanted, intrusive, unacceptable, and persistent thought, image, or impulse. Obsessions are not voluntarily produced, but are experienced as events that interrupt one's attention. The affected person recognizes that these thoughts are his own, and are not introduced or controlled by some outer force or other person. This is an important feature since, in certain mental illnesses, patients may feel that thoughts have been inserted into their heads by other people, outside agents, or even by the radio or TV. Obsessions are not experienced in this way. The thoughts can be repugnant, blasphemous, obscene, worrying, nonsensical, or all of these. The person neither wants nor welcomes them; instead, he resists them and tries to get rid of them. They are characteristically difficult to block or suppress, and at times the sufferer feels besieged by them (the word 'obsession' is derived from the Latin '*obsidere*', to be besieged). They are intrusive as well as tenacious. The person may be engaged in some activity, such as driving a car or trying to study, when the obsession intrudes into his consciousness. It interrupts his ordinary, preferred thinking and behaviour.

Virtually all obsessions clash with the person's important values and are unacceptable, shameful, repugnant, and upsetting. They give rise to painful self-doubting.

Some examples of obsessions are as follows:

- A 25-year-old woman had recurrent intrusive impulses to strangle domestic animals. They were followed by the thought or doubt that she might actually have done so.

- A woman had recurrent intrusive thoughts that she was contaminated by dirt and germs from strangers or, worse, that she was inadvertently contaminating other people.

- A man had recurrent intrusive doubts that he might have driven into a pedestrian, and often felt compelled to retrace his journey to check.

- A trainee nurse was tormented by recurrent thoughts that she might lose control one day and sexually molest a child.

- A young man had the recurrent intrusive thought 'Christ was a bastard'. He also felt an impulse to shout this out during a church service.

- A woman had the recurrent intrusive thought that she might offend people by touching them in a sexual, inappropriate manner.

- An engineer had recurrent intrusive images of himself violently attacking his parents with a kitchen knife. The obsession included images of the victims, of blood flowing, and of injuries caused.

- A woman had recurrent, intrusive impulses to harm herself by damaging her eyes. They were accompanied by vivid images of the act.

- A 14-year-old girl had recurrent impulses to blurt out nasty obscenities in public. She had tormenting doubts about whether or not she had already done so.

- An occupational therapist had recurrent thoughts that she might harm cyclists by pushing them into busy traffic.

Obsessions occur in one of three forms: a thought, an image, or an impulse, or a combination of these. When the obsession intrudes, the person usually resists it. Even if he succeeds in blocking it, it is likely to return within a short period of time. Some patients report that their obsessions are with them most of their waking hours, despite desperate struggles to get rid of them. The mental effort involved in attempting to subdue obsessions can be exhausting, even though the struggle is not evident to friends and relatives. For some it feels as if the obsession is always there, lurking at the back of their minds.

Obsessions tend to flourish during periods of unoccupied solitude, and are less frequent during pleasant conversations or other engaging activities.

Different uses of the word 'obsession'

The meaning of the technical term 'obsession' in the context of obsessive–compulsive disorder is different from its meaning in day-to-day language. We often hear someone being described as 'obsessional about his job', and expressions such as, 'He is obsessed with her', 'Football is an obsession with him', and so on. What is meant in such instances is that the person in question has an unusually great interest in something or someone, spends a lot of time thinking about it, and can become preoccupied. But such an attachment, interest, or preoccupation is not seen by him as unwanted or unacceptable, and there is no resistance, nor any attempt to block it. These preoccupations are pleasing and welcome, and are promoted unless they occur at inconvenient times. They are very different from the way the clinical, technical term 'obsession' is used in reference to the unwanted and unwelcome intrusive thoughts that occur in obsessive–compulsive disorders.

Features of obsessions

What are the contents of obsessions? There are three common themes, in descending order of frequency: unwanted thoughts of aggression/harm, unwanted sexual thoughts, and blasphemous thoughts. The harm obsessions are the most common, and the blasphemous ones are the least common.

These are examples of obsessions with an aggression/harm theme. The person repeatedly has unwanted, unwelcome thoughts of harming elderly people, say by pushing them in front of oncoming traffic, or of attacking or molesting children. Obsessions often produce a fear of losing control—'What if one day I lose control and attack an elderly person?'. Sexual obsessions often include recurrent images, as well as thoughts of repugnant unacceptable sexual wishes or acts, such as incestuous thoughts, molesting children, and images of sexual exhibitionism. As with the aggressive obsessions, those with sexual content often arouse a fear of losing control, which in turn leads to avoidance of the people or places that are associated with the obsessions. People who experience recurrent intrusive thoughts of molesting children generally take great care to avoid being alone with a child. Blasphemous obsessions, such as having obscene thoughts about sacred figures or shrines, can be extremely upsetting and give rise to tormenting self-doubt and self-criticism. 'I must be a total hypocrite to have these recurrent thoughts while appearing to be a righteous and religious person.'

It is probable that obsessions develop when the affected person mistakenly attaches great personal significance to the uninvited and repugnant thoughts that virtually everyone experiences from time to time (see pp. 14–15). Whereas most people dismiss these thoughts as nonsensical and insignificant, some extremely sensitive people with highly elevated personal standards regard them as being important. If the affected person interprets the intrusive thoughts as being personally revealing and highly significant, then they tend to recur over and over again.

There is a strong tendency to conceal these recurrent and repugnant thoughts, mainly because the affected person anticipates, usually incorrectly, that if other people learn about these thoughts they too would interpret them as being revealing and highly significant. 'If other people really knew about my ugly thoughts they would recoil and brand me a monster.' One patient described his aggressive and sexual obsessions as 'my ugly little secret'. The mistaken interpretations made by patients who are tormented by obsessions generally lead to one or all of these conclusions about their 'deep, true character'—it means that 'I am mad, bad, or dangerous, or all three of these'.

Senseless and trivial obsessions, such as advertising jingles, are rare but can be a troublesome nuisance. In some cases, the obsession consists of a doubting thought, which can apply to most things that the person does. For example, a young woman complained that, whenever she performed any action, she would immediately be assailed by the thought 'Did I do it right?' or 'Have I done the right thing?'.

Obsessions produce internal resistance, which can take various forms such as trying to block the thought/image/impulse, endlessly debating with oneself, praying repeatedly, trying to neutralize or wipe out the thoughts, or even escaping completely from the situation in which the thought is experienced. Obsessions can also lead the patient to avoid other people.

Thought–action fusion

In some instances, an intrusive thought becomes significant because of a tendency to regard thoughts as being psychologically equivalent to the corresponding action. Thus, having the thought 'I may strangle someone' is regarded as being as reprehensible as actually strangling a person; there is a moral equivalence. A related tendency is to believe that, because one has had a thought about a misfortune or disaster, the likelihood of that misfortune actually occurring is increased. A university student was extremely disturbed by recurring intrusive images of his parents in a motor vehicle accident because he felt that his images actually increased the probability that they would have an accident. If a patient attaches great significance to this form of 'biased' thinking, termed 'thought–action fusion', he feels responsible for potentially harming someone else, and the ensuing guilt and distress add to his problems.

What are compulsions?

A compulsion is purposeful, meaningful, and deliberate behaviour that the person feels driven to carry out repeatedly, and is usually performed according to certain rules or in a stereotyped fashion. The aim is to prevent harm or misfortunes occurring to oneself or others. For example, a patient attempts to remove some contamination by washing his hands over and over again in order to prevent an illness. Another patient feels compelled to check the safety of the front door a dozen times in order to prevent a burglary. The act is preceded or accompanied by a sense of subjective compulsion—i.e. the person feels a powerful urge to engage in the preventive behaviour. Patients who wash compulsively can damage the skin on their hands, and, in an extreme case, a patient continued washing his hands in hot water despite traces of blood in the wash-basin.

In most instances the person recognizes the senselessness or irrationality of the behaviour. The behaviour is regarded as appropriate but excessive or overelaborate. There is a desire to bring the checking/washing behaviour down to a realistic level, but the urge repeatedly to do it 'thoroughly' is over-powering. No pleasure is derived from carrying it out, although it can provide a release of tension or a feeling of relief in the short term.

The most common compulsions involve repeated and stereotyped washing or checking:

◆ A woman repeatedly and extensively washed her hands to get rid of contamination by germs. The washing was done in an elaborate ritual, six times without soap and six times with soap, on each occasion.

- A young man checked door handles, gas taps, and electric switches every time he went past them.

- An accountant had to check his calculations dozens and dozens of times. As a result he worked 12-hour days but was always behind and had to give up the job.

- A 15-year-old girl cleaned and washed the area around her bed, including the wall, every night before going to bed, in order to rid it of germs and dirt.

- A man opened letters he had written and sealed, to make sure that he had written the correct things. He would rip open the envelope, re-read the letter, and put it into a new one, several times before posting it. A contemporary form of this compulsion is repeatedly checking one's e-mail messages, over and over again, before sending them, or simply deleting them.

- A woman who feared that she might develop cancer checked her body up to 10 times per day.

- A man had the compulsion to touch with the left hand anything he had touched with the right hand, and vice versa.

- A man with an intense fear of dirt felt compelled to shower at least six times per day, always washing his body in the same stereotyped manner.

- A woman had the compulsion to wipe, with a wet cloth, all tables and worktops several times, each time that she was to use them. She did this to get rid of what she called 'invisible food particles'.

- A manager spent at least an hour repeatedly checking all the windows and doors of his store before leaving for home; members of the staff were able to carry out the same procedure in 5 minutes.

- A 35-year-old married woman had the compulsion to wash and disinfect herself and her clothes, out of fear of contracting cancer. She spent many hours each day doing this.

The person feels an irresistible urge—compulsive urge—to engage in a particular behaviour, which he carries out repeatedly despite recognizing that it is irrational or excessive. The avowed purpose is to prevent a misfortune or avoid harm, and the person feels a special responsibility for these preventive acts.

Compulsive cleaning

The driving force behind most cases of compulsive cleaning is an intense fear of contamination. The purpose of the repetitive washing/cleaning is to remove the threat of the perceived contamination.

Feelings of contamination fall into two main categories. In the most common form, the person feels contaminated by physical contact with dangerous, dirty, or disgusting objects or materials (e.g. dirty needles, chemicals, decaying food, urine, faeces). A second type of contamination, mental contamination, can arise from actual or indirect associations with people who are believed to have harmed the patient in some way.

Contamination is an intense, persisting, and unpleasant feeling of having been polluted or infected by physical contact with, or by association with, a place or person that is soiled, impure, infectious—or a combination of these. Contamination is accompanied by unpleasant emotions, among which fear, disgust, guilt, immorality, and shame are prominent. Feelings of contamination instigate vigorous attempts to remove, to clean away, the infectious material, the dirt, the impurity. Intensive, meticulous, repetitive washing and cleaning compulsions are undertaken in an attempt to remove the feeling of dirtiness and protect one's health. As a secondary consequence, it leads to extensive avoidance of situations in which the person fears that there is the possibility of contact with a contaminant. In extreme cases, patients avoid entire 'contaminated' cities. Public washrooms are a great problem; they are perceived to be particularly threatening, and if it is impossible totally to avoid them, then patients adopt a variety of rudimentary protective measures, such as opening the doors with their feet or elbows, using a Kleenex, or walking in behind another person. Some patients feel that their contamination can be transmitted to other people and will go to great lengths to avoid spreading it.

We are all familiar with the feeling of contamination that arises when we touch something dirty or polluted, and we are equally familiar with the resulting urge to wash away the contaminant. In patients with obsessive–compulsive disorder, the sensitivity to actual or perceived contamination is heightened, the feelings are extremely intense, and the anticipated consequences are catastrophic. This is the familiar form of contamination after physical contact with a pollutant. The less familiar form of mental contamination can be equally distressing and damaging but is far less obvious.

Compulsive cleaning is one of the most common, classical, manifestations of obsessive–compulsive disorder.

Checking compulsions

Checking compulsions are attempts to reduce the probability of some misfortune occurring; patients repeatedly check the safety of electrical appliances, doors, vehicles, and check their work repeatedly if they believe that an error might have serious consequences. The urges to check and re-check are driven by an inflated sense of responsibility for protecting others and oneself from catastrophic errors or carelessness. An experienced pharmacist who worked in a large pharmacy had prepared over 10 000 prescriptions during the past 10 years. He had made only two trivial errors in that period, but every day went to work expecting that he might make a serious error. He estimated that the probability of such an error, every working day, was 100%. He estimated the probability of equally experienced colleagues making an error as 0.001%. He rated his own probable 'error' as totally catastrophic, probably fatal, but a colleague's error as minor. At the same time he felt that he was at least as competent as most of his colleagues, and superior to many of them.

A grossly inflated sense of personal responsibility is present in most cases of compulsive checking and, as illustrated above, is combined with inflated estimates of the probability of making an error and inflated expectations of the seriousness of the feared error. It is not surprising that certain jobs are a trial for patients with a tendency to check repeatedly; they include pharmacy, law, accountancy, medicine, security officers, safety inspectors, and so on.

As with washing compulsions, the affected people feel that their checking behaviour is appropriate but excessive, out of control and damaging. Moreover, even when they have completed their actual checking rituals, they continue to check mentally. They are never off-duty mentally. It is a draining and endlessly frustrating, exhausting problem.

Covert compulsions

Many patients have covert compulsions that have the features of observable compulsions:

♦ A man had the compulsion to say silently a string of specific 'safe' words whenever he heard or read of any disaster or accident.

♦ A woman, who was distressed by the recurrent intrusion of unwelcome and obscene words, carried out a compulsion each time this happened. She tried with little success to deal with the obsessions by changing the words into similar but acceptable ones—e.g. 'well' for 'hell'—and saying them silently four times.

- A middle-aged man had the compulsion to visualize everything that was said to him and could not reply until he had formed these visual images. Often this would take time, leading to long silences that were puzzling to others.

- A woman, who was tormented by intrusive repetitions of bloody images of her relations and friends, felt compelled to re-constitute the images until the people concerned appeared to be in good health. This method of trying to deal with such images, re-animation, is not uncommon among patients suffering from recurrent violent/harmful images.

- A woman became very worried if she set her eyes on black objects, especially if this occurred immediately before retiring to bed. When this happened she had the obsessional thought that it would cause her to go blind, or lead to some other disaster. So every time she experienced the thought, she felt compelled to neutralize the obsession by visualizing an object of a different colour, usually white, as a way of preventing disaster.

- A woman who had the recurrent obsessional thought that she was responsible for any murders that she read or heard about engaged in the compulsion of silently saying 'I did not do it' seven times, each time such a thought came.

The active nature of compulsions

It needs to be stressed that compulsions are actively carried out, and for a recognized purpose. *Compulsions are not mere repetitions*; they are purposeful, meaningful, and deliberate behaviour. The patient is not happy about doing it, but it is a voluntary and controllable action that is performed reluctantly, almost against their wishes. The urges driving the compulsions are strong but the compulsive behaviour can be partly controlled—it can be postponed, it can be lengthened, partly abbreviated, re-shaped, concealed, and, in certain circumstances, it can be carried out for the patient by another person (e.g. checking behaviour). The malleability of the compulsive behaviour is most evident in compulsive checking—it can be lengthened, abbreviated, postponed, often concealed, and so on. Compulsions are driven but they are not totally inflexible, and they are not automatic behaviour. They are different from the tics and muscle spasms that are observed in some people, especially children, which are essentially involuntary, meaningless, purposeless, repetitive motor responses. These are not actively, deliberately carried out by the patient, and are not compulsions.

Sometimes the mere occurrence of repetitive behaviour is mistaken for the compulsive behaviour seen in obsessive–compulsive disorders. This can be a source of confusion but is easily clarified when a full psychological assessment is carried out.

Resistance

Obsessions and compulsions are generally resisted. For some time it was considered by many experts that resistance is an essential feature of obsessive–compulsive disorders, but there are exceptions. In the majority of cases, the person does resist the obsession or the compulsive urge, especially in the early stages of the disorder. However, after repeated failures effectively to resist the obsessions and compulsions, the person's resistance may wane. Patients with strongly established, chronic obsessive–compulsive problems may report little or no resistance to the obsessions or the compulsive urges because they have yielded to them.

Different uses of the word 'compulsion'

As with the term 'obsession', our use of the clinical, technical term 'compulsion' is different from, and more specific than, the way it is used in everyday language. It is common to hear about 'compulsive lying', 'compulsive eating', 'compulsive gambling', and so on. These types of behaviour are different from the kinds of clinical compulsions that we are concerned with here. As noted, compulsions are repetitive acts that are the result of an urge, which the person usually tries to resist, and which are carried out reluctantly. They are seen as essentially irrational or senseless, and give no pleasure or satisfaction. Forms of behaviour such as compulsive eating and gambling do not show these features—although they are problems in their own right, they are not indicative of an obsessive–compulsive disorder.

Sometimes the term 'compulsive' is used for behaviour such as recurrent nail-biting, thumb-sucking, and hair-pulling. These are habits, and the person usually engages in them, at least part of the time, without being aware of them. They lack the characteristic features of the compulsion in obsessive–compulsive disorder, such as purposefulness and meaningfulness, and certainly cannot be performed for the person by someone else. True compulsions are carried out in order to accomplish some aim; behaviours such as nail-biting, hair-pulling, and so on are not, and nor do they provoke a feeling of resistance. These kinds of behaviour are best seen as habits rather than true compulsions, as their similarity to the latter is superficial.

Putting matters right

Some instances of compulsive behaviour are attempts to 'put matters right'—for example, to ensure that one's appearance is exactly right, to place one's belongings in a particular place, or ordered in a rigidly prescribed manner:

A 28-year-old man spent up to 5 hours per day combing and brushing his hair 'to get it right', and felt extremely uncomfortable till he succeeded. Whenever he left his home he wore a cap to conceal his hair, unless it felt perfectly right.

The urge to put matters right is associated with the compulsion to arrange and order one's possessions (books, clothes, papers). This can take many hours and must be satisfactorily completed before leaving or before starting on a fresh task. Intense ordering and arranging is more noticeable in child obsessive–compulsive disorder than in adult cases, perhaps because other, and more severe, compulsions arise in adulthood and overshadow the compulsion to order and arrange. People, young or old, who feel compelled to introduce and maintain inflexible order can react strongly if their 'systems' are disrupted. The drive for order can be associated with the comparable compulsion to introduce symmetry and exact balances, mainly pertaining to one's possessions.

A self-report scale for assessing the compulsions to order, arrange, and ensure symmetry, is reproduced in Appendix 5.

The diagnosis of obsessive–compulsive disorder

A person may be considered to have an obsessive–compulsive disorder if he experiences or displays obsessions or compulsions, or both. However, it is necessary to add an important qualification: it is not merely the presence of obsessions and/or compulsions as such that matters, but the degree to which they cause distress and/or interfere with the person's life. As mentioned earlier, it is customary to grade the seriousness of the disorder, from 'mild' to 'moderate' or 'severe'.

As a result of recent publicity there is a tendency to over-diagnose obsessive–compulsive disorders. For example, in a study carried out in Canada in 1997, clear indications of over-diagnoses were obtained. After a 'screening' for the disorder in a community sample, a full clinical assessment revealed that well over half of the provisional diagnoses of obsessive–compulsive disorder were incorrect. Numbers of people who reported troubling worries or repetitive behaviour were initially over-diagnosed, but in the subsequent comprehensive clinical examinations no significant symptoms of obsessive–compulsive disorder were detected. There were many 'false positives'. For this reason it is essential to ensure that the person receives a full and accurate assessment.

Obsessions and compulsions in the general population

It is important to recognize that obsessions and compulsions are not uncommon in the general population. There are many people who have mild versions of obsessions and/or compulsions, but never go to a clinic or hospital seeking help.

Normal obsessions

Research studies carried out in different countries have shown that many people, randomly selected from the general population, in fact about four-fifths of them, report experiencing unwanted, unwelcome, even repugnant intrusive thoughts. These intrusions are similar in form and content to the obsessions of patients who seek help. The differences are that the non-patients tend to have the unwelcome intrusions far less frequently, are seldom distressed by them, and can easily dismiss them. In a study that was carried out in London some years ago, we asked a random sample of people to tell us if they ever experienced any unwelcome, objectionable, repugnant, and intrusive thoughts. These are some of the intrusions that they described:

- impulse to harm innocent people (e.g. children, elderly people);

- impulse to shout obscenities in church;

- thoughts of 'unnatural' sexual acts;

- thoughts of driving into pedestrians;

- images of her parents lying dead;

- objectionable sexual thoughts and images while attempting to pray;

- impulse to disrupt the peace at a gathering (e.g. shout or throw things);

- impulse to expose oneself;

- impulse to attack violently and kill a dog;

- sexual thoughts about religious figures, e.g. the Virgin Mary.

The content of the intrusions was similar to the obsessions commonly reported by obsessive–compulsive patients.

Normal compulsions

Similarly, a large proportion of people have normal 'compulsions'. Various forms of checking behaviour are commonplace. Consider, for example, a person who goes round the house several times in order to make sure that all gas taps are closed, before leaving home; or a person who returns to the kitchen three or four times to check that the oven is switched off. Many people have minor compulsive rituals, such as always putting on the left shoe first, or always arranging a desk in a rigidly unchanging way. Studies have shown that such minor compulsions are common in the general population.

An excellent account of an eccentric non-clinical compulsion is provided in Boswell's biography of Samuel Johnson, the great eighteenth-century man of letters. Boswell described various 'singularities' or 'particularities' of Johnson's behaviour:

'He had another particularity, of which none of his friends ever ventured to ask an explanation. It appeared to be some superstitious habit, which he had contracted early, and from which he had never called upon his reason to disentangle him. This was his anxious care to go out or in at a door or passage by a certain number of steps from a certain point, or at least so as that either his right or his left foot (I am not certain which) should constantly make the first actual movement when he came close to the door or passage. Thus I conjecture: for I have upon innumerable occasions, observed him suddenly stop, and then seem to count his steps with a deep earnestness; and when he had neglected or gone wrong in this sort of magical movement, I have seen him go back again, put himself in a proper position to begin the ceremony, and, having gone through it, break from his abstraction, walk briskly on, and join his companion.'

Superstitions

There are similarities between superstitious ideas and some obsessions, and between superstitious acts and compulsive behaviour. Superstitions and certain obsessions are similar in that the person recognizes the irrationality of the idea or its associated activity, but prefers to err on the side of caution or safety. Like compulsions, many superstitious acts are carried out in order to prevent a misfortune from happening. However, there are many superstitious acts that are carried out in order to enhance the probability of good fortune; this is never the case with compulsive behaviour. Furthermore, obsessions can be distinguished from most superstitions in that the content of the obsession is often unacceptable or repugnant, leads to resistance, and causes distress. Obsessions are uniquely personal, whereas superstitions tend to be shared by many members of one's community or family.

Superstitions in children are discussed in Chapter 9.

Distress and interference

In deciding whether a diagnosis of obsessive–compulsive disorder is appropriate, it is essential to assess whether the person is significantly distressed by the obsessions and/or compulsions and whether they impair his normal functioning. Experiencing an unwanted thought once a day is unlikely to cause distress, but if it recurs dozens of times every hour it will be distressing and damaging. Similarly, checking all the gas taps once or twice before leaving home causes neither impairment nor distress, but if one were to check, say, 10 times on each occasion, that would interfere with one's normal functioning. Some patients reach clinics or hospitals only after the problem has progressed to such a degree that it produces drastic effects on their lives. For example, a woman came for help only when her compulsions had developed to such an extent that she was spending all her waking hours cleaning the house. Another patient gave up his job because he was increasingly fearful that he would pick up dangerous germs from contact with other people

Sometimes the person's obsessions and compulsions are more distressing to others than to himself. For example, a man who was excessively concerned about germs and dirt carried out intensive washing and cleaning compulsions. This might never have become a problem in itself, but he began to insist that his wife and mother-in-law did the same. If they refused he would get angry with them, and insisted that they both wash their hands at specified times, that they keep their towels only in designated safe places, and so on. The initial distress was felt not by him, but by those who were living with him.

In some, the compulsion is a minor one that does not affect one's life or functioning ordinarily, but can be a problem in certain circumstances. A 26-year-old man had the compulsion to look at any stranger a second time. If he noticed someone on the street who went past him, he would immediately turn round and look at the person a second time. This was a harmless if peculiar compulsion, and remained so until he developed a relationship with a woman. She noticed this behaviour and inferred that he was showing an unhealthy interest in other women, despite the fact that he was looking at members of both sexes indiscriminately. The ensuing dispute nearly caused the break-up of their relationship. This problem brought him to a psychologist for advice; otherwise he might never have felt any need to seek help. In another case, a man was accosted by store detectives in a large supermarket. He admitted that he had acted in a way that might have given rise to suspicion. He explained that he had a compulsion to touch with one hand anything that he had touched with the other, even if he had to turn round and go back to the object to do so, and to make the hand in question free by transferring whatever he was carrying to his other hand. Until the embarrassing event, he had not realized what a spectacle he was making of himself in public places.

Unwelcome intrusive thoughts, even mild obsessions and compulsions, are common among people in the general population, and are not considered to be problems unless they cause distress or interfere with one's life. If a person experiences obsessions and/or compulsions that cause distress, or seriously affect his life, professional advice should be considered.

The matter needs to be kept in perspective. Only a small minority of people suffer from diagnosable obsessive–compulsive disorder, and, as noted, there is a tendency for the disorder to be over-diagnosed.

The relationship between obsessions and compulsions

Thus far, obsessions and compulsions have been discussed as separate phenomena. What is the relationship between them? In some of the examples of compulsions given above, a relationship between the two is clearly implied. In many cases the recurrent obsession drives the compulsive behaviour. We referred, for instance, to a woman who had recurrent intrusive thoughts (obsession) that she might go blind whenever she saw black objects, which led to her engaging in the compulsive mental activity of visualizing objects of different colours (see p. 11). To give a common example, when someone gets the obsessional thought that he might have touched something that contaminated him, he is likely to feel a strong urge to decontaminate himself by compulsively washing his hands repeatedly. These compulsions are sometimes described as 'neutralizing' behaviour because they 'put right' the disturbance caused by the obsession; they serve to neutralize the disturbance and/or threat. Many people try to neutralize their obsessional images, and learn by trial and error which tactics help them. They include attempts to substitute an acceptable image, or attempts to mask the intrusive image, and some people try to control them by blocking their eyes or blinking rapidly. These attempts at neutralizing seldom provide patients with more than brief relief. However, it is probable that many people who experience non-clinical obsessional images develop successful methods for coping with them, by neutralizing or other means.

Obsessions do not necessarily provoke compulsions; in many instances they generate and sustain avoidance behaviour. For example, avoidance behaviour is a common reaction to obsessional thoughts about sexual molestation.

In the large majority of cases of compulsive washing the driving force is a fear of contamination, and any actual or perceived contact with a contaminant will trigger the urge to wash/clean. Most commonly, checking compulsions are triggered by a perceived need to prevent accidents or misfortunes; these compulsions tend to occur in familiar situations at home or work, and are remarkably limited in range.

There are cases in which a compulsion recurs without any preceding obsession, as in the following example.

> A man had a compulsion to imagine car registration plates in a certain way. Every time he noticed a car licence number plate, he compulsively visualized the same plate with the number transformed in certain specific ways, such as squared, halved, or multiplied by two.

Many people with extensive touching compulsions do not report accompanying or preceding obsessions. Obsessions play little or no part in compulsive hoarding or in primary obsessional slowness (p. 59).

Elements of an obsessive–compulsive experience

The relationship between obsessions and compulsions can be illustrated by considering the elements that may be present in an obsessive–compulsive experience (Table 1.3).

Table 1.3 Elements of an obsessive–compulsive experience

Trigger	external/internal/none
Obsession	thought/image/impulse/none
Discomfort	+
Compulsive urge	+/−

Table 1.3 Elements of an obsessive–compulsive experience (*continued*)

Compulsive behaviour	motor/cognitive/none
Reduction of discomfort	+/?
Fear of disaster	+/−
Inflated responsibility	+/−
Reassurance seeking	+/−
Avoidance	+/−
Disruption	external/internal/none

+ Indicates 'present'; − indicates 'absent'.

Trigger

A trigger is an event, or a cue, that sets off an obsession, a feeling or discomfort, or indeed a compulsive urge. A trigger may be external—i.e. something in the environment—or internal. For example, a young woman had the obsession 'Did I stab someone?' or 'Will I stab my children?' every time she saw a knife or any other sharp object: the knife was the external trigger that provoked her obsession. Internal triggers are mental events that lead to the same result. A man complained that every time he remembered his deceased father, he experienced distressing obsessions about death. The memory of the father was the internal trigger for his obsessional thoughts. As indicated in Table 1.3, triggers are not invariably present in all obsessive–compulsive experiences.

Discomfort

The occurrence of an obsession usually produces a feeling of discomfort. For many, this feeling is best described as anxiety, but some patients report that what they feel is not anxiety, but general unease, tension, or even a sense of guilt. 'Discomfort' is thus a preferred term because it encompasses all these emotions. Note that Table 1.3 states that obsessive–compulsive experiences always include discomfort; this may, however, not be so for non-clinical instances.

Compulsive urge

This is the urge, or drive, that the person feels to carry out a 'prescribed' behaviour, usually in order to reduce his discomfort. As Table 1.3 shows, not every obsessive–compulsive experience has this element.

Compulsive behaviour

This is the behaviour, overt or covert, that results from the compulsive urge. When the term 'compulsion' is used, it usually refers to the compulsive urge and the compulsive behaviour taken together.

Reduction of discomfort/anxiety

When the compulsive behaviour is carried out in the required manner, the patient normally feels relieved; the discomfort caused by the obsession (and/ or the trigger, and/or the compulsive urge) is reduced or eliminated. Table 1.3 has included a question mark against this element of obsessive–compulsive experience. This is because there are instances in which carrying out the compulsive behaviour does not lead to a reduction of discomfort. Indeed, in a small number of cases the discomfort may even increase. Moreover, even when the compulsive behaviour reduces the anxiety or discomfort, the person may be left feeling frustrated and demoralized.

Fear of disaster

These fears arise frequently. The patient feels that a disaster will happen unless he neutralizes it by carrying out his compulsive behaviour. For example, an elderly man had the very strong fear that, if he did not check the gas taps in his house a certain number of times, the house would explode and go up in flames. The relationship between the specific disaster feared and the compulsive behaviour is, of course, not always logical. For example, a young man felt that his hand-washing compulsions prevented accidents occurring to his family members who lived in a different country. Similarly, patients who are troubled by fears of contamination, such as contracting AIDS, may wash excessively even though they know that washing your hands is not an effective precaution against AIDS.

Inflated responsibility

Many patients experience an inflated sense of responsibility—even for events over which they have no control. This is particularly common among those whose main problem is excessive checking. The inflated responsibility commonly generates anxiety and guilt.

Most examples of compulsive checking are attempts to prevent a misfortune, however obscure. The person strives for certainty that no harm will occur to others because of his negligence or supposedly poor memory. 'I must check at least ten times to be absolutely sure that the stove is off and will not cause a deadly fire.' The drive to check repeatedly is intensified if, and when, the person feels solely or largely responsible for safety; for example, if they are the last person to leave the house or office. Curiously, there is a tendency for affected people to believe that an accident or misfortune is definitely more likely to occur when they are responsible for the task than when someone else is responsible. This is one example of the so-called 'cognitive biases', or skewed reasoning, that often occur in obsessive–compulsive disorders.

This is a selection of the ideas and feelings reported by people with inflated responsibility:

◆ 'I feel anxious and guilty if I have not made absolutely sure that my family and friends are safe';

◆ 'I feel especially responsible for checking the safety of my home and workplace—far more than my family and colleagues';

◆ 'If I have not repeatedly checked the total safety of my home, I feel uneasy and very reluctant to leave';

◆ 'I definitely feel responsible for constantly protecting my family and friends—I am always on duty'.

Inflated feelings of responsibility make such a large contribution to obsessive–compulsive disorders that some sufferers try to fend off responsibilities; for example, by refusing promotions to more responsible positions. They are likely to be distressed if their responsibilities are increased, and for this reason avoid such increases at work and home. However, a reasoned and reasonable transfer of responsibility for therapeutic purposes can be a great relief.

Reassurance seeking

Many obsessive–compulsive patients resort to reassurance seeking, usually from members of their families. Often, obsessional thoughts such as 'Will I go insane?', 'Did I do it properly?', and 'Do I need to check the taps again?' lead to the patient repeatedly asking for reassurance. When reassurance is received, the patient feels some brief relief from his discomfort, but the doubts and anxiety soon return. Frequently repeated requests for reassurance, often using the same words or phrases over and over again, strain the patience of friends and family.

In many instances, the requests for reassurance are not actually requests for information, despite the form of the question. The patient knows full well what the answer to his question really is. What seems to be a request for information is instead an indirect attempt to reduce his anxiety.

Avoidance

This can be a significant factor in the clinical picture, although it is not part of the obsessive–compulsive experience as such, but rather a consequence of the obsessive–compulsive disorder. Usually, the avoidance behaviour concerns objects and situations that might trigger or exacerbate the obsession or compulsion. Those who fear contamination from dirt and germs strive to avoid what they believe to be any potential source of germs, be it a place or a person. Those with checking compulsions avoid tasks or situations that will increase their sense of responsibility and/or might be unsafe. A woman who had the obsessional thought that she might stab her children went to great lengths to avoid contact with knives, scissors, and other sharp objects. A man, who feared that he might catch AIDS, totally avoided certain areas of London.

A married woman in her twenties had the recurring thought that she had cancer. After several years of checking for cancer symptoms, she began to avoid any situation where she feared she might discover she had signs of cancer. She would not make her bed in the morning, or look at her used underwear, for fear of discovering blood stains which, to her, would be a sign of the dreaded illness. She even stopped looking at herself in the mirror or at her own body. She began to wear blouses and jumpers with long sleeves so that she could not see her arms, and trousers so that she could not see her legs. She stopped washing herself properly, as she feared that she might discover lumps on her body.

In some cases, certain 'unsafe' numbers, letters, or colours are avoided because the patient feels that such avoidance is necessary in order to avert some disaster, usually to a loved one. An illustration of this is found in the following example.

A married woman began to avoid the number four. Her husband's birthday was on the fourth day of the month and her obsessional logic dictated that, if she failed to avoid the number, she would cause great harm to him. She went to great lengths to avoid the number; for instance, she would skip the fourth page of books and magazines she was reading, would never write the number four, never eat four of anything (e.g. potatoes or slices of bread), and so on. Life became impossible when this gradually extended to all numbers beginning or ending with four, multiples of four, those that are adjacent to four, and so on, at which point she sought help.

Disruption

When an obsessive–compulsive patient engages in his compulsion, he needs to carry it out precisely as he feels it ought to be done. If the behaviour is disrupted, the compulsive ritual is invalidated and needs to be restarted. For long and complicated rituals this can be extremely time-consuming and exhausting. The events that can act as disruptors vary from noise and other external disturbances to certain classes of experiences and thoughts, or the presence of other people. Hence, many compulsions—checking and/or cleaning—are carried out privately, when alone at night.

> A middle-aged man had recurrent, intrusive thoughts and images of past homosexual experiences. This led to feelings of guilt and distress, and he felt compelled to 'cleanse his mind' with silent prayers to God, uttered in a certain fixed sequence. If, during this praying, images of homosexual acts arose in his mind, he had to restart the praying.

The need to form a safe or suitable thought before carrying out a compulsive or other act is common. If the action is disturbed by an unacceptable thought, the compulsive sequence has to be repeated in full.

> A man engaged in prolonged hand-washing rituals whenever he felt his hands were contaminated by dirt and germs. He would usually wash them at the kitchen sink. If, during the activity, he happened to catch a glimpse of the kitchen waste bin, which he considered to be a dirty object, he felt his washing was not effective. So he would restart the washing ritual.

In some instances the person feels compelled to clear his mind by removing all other thoughts before attempting to carry out the compulsive activity; for example, removing distracting thoughts, all the better to concentrate on making sure that you have checked the stove correctly. Patients who carry out compulsive checking tend to lose confidence in their memory and in their ability to concentrate, especially when they are checking.

Other terms and concepts

There are two other key terms, which are commonly used to describe aspects of obsessive–compulsive disorder that need explanation. They are 'ritual' and 'rumination'.

What is a ritual?

A ritual is a compulsion that is carried out in a rigid, set pattern, and a sequence of steps with a clear beginning and end. The following example illustrates an elaborate ritual reported by a man in his mid-twenties.

- Enter bathroom with left foot first.

- Close door with left hand, then touch door handle with right hand.

- Take towel from rail and keep it on edge of bath with left hand, then touch it with right hand.

- Take toothbrush from cabinet and place it on edge of wash-basin with left hand, then touch it with right hand.

- Take toothpaste tube from cabinet with left hand, then touch it with right hand.

- Unscrew and remove cap with left hand, then touch it with right hand.

- Squeeze tube to get enough toothpaste on to brush with left hand, then touch tube with right hand.

- Replace cap of tube with left hand, then touch it with right hand.

- Put tube back with left hand, then touch it with right hand.

- Pick up brush with left hand, then start brushing: teeth brushed in twos, from left to right, top row first, bottom row next, outside first, inside next, each set of two eight times; then, repeat whole process with brush in right hand, then again with left hand followed by same again with right hand.

- Open taps with left hand, then touch them with right hand.

- Wash brush under hot tap, held in left hand, then touch it with right hand.

- Put brush back in cabinet with left hand, then touch it with right hand.

- Rinse mouth, taking water with left hand, then with right hand.

- Look at self in mirror first with left eye, then with right eye.

- Begin to wash face, using left hand to splash water on face, then right hand.

- Rub left side of face with left hand, followed by right side of face with left hand, then rub left side of face with right hand, followed by right side of face with right hand.

- Apply soap to face, in the same sequence as above.

- Rinse face, splashing water on face with left hand, then with right hand.

- Look at self in the mirror, first with left eye, them with right eye.

- Close taps with left hand, then touch them with right hand.

- Pick up towel with left hand, then touch it with right hand.

- Dry face with towel, left side holding towel in left hand, then right side holding towel in left hand, then left side holding towel in right hand, then right side holding towel in right hand.

- Look at self in mirror, first with left eye, then with right eye.

- Put towel back on rail with left hand, then touch it with right hand.

- Open door with left hand, then touch handle with right hand.

- Leave bathroom, with left foot first.

What are ruminations?

A rumination is a train of thought about a question or theme that is undirected, unproductive, and prolonged. Unlike obsessions, ruminations are not objectionable repugnant intrusions and are not resisted. During a rumination, the person appears to be deeply occupied, very thoughtful, and detached. Some authors and clinicians use the term 'obsessional rumination' to refer to all obsessional thoughts, but this is misleading. An example of a rumination is as follows:

> A young man had complicated and time-consuming rumination on the question: 'Is everyone basically good?'. He would ruminate on this for a long time, going over in his mind various considerations and arguments, and contemplating what superficially appeared to him to be relevant evidence. This never led to a solution or satisfactory conclusion.

How does a rumination differ from an obsession? Many ruminations of obsessive–compulsive patients dwell on religious, philosophical, or metaphysical topics, such as the origins of the universe, life after death, the nature of morality, and so on. They are not unpleasant and are indulged rather than resisted. They rarely cause distress and are not disabling.

Unlike obsessions, ruminations are not clearly circumscribed, and they drift along rather than intrude into the patient's consciousness. Ruminations are not well-defined events; the theme or the question of the rumination is discernible, but the process of thinking about the topic is diffuse, often rambling, and open-ended.

One young man reported extensive ruminations about what would happen to him after death. He would weigh up the various theoretical possibilities, visualize scenes of heaven, hell, and other worlds, try to remember what philosophers and scientists have said about death, and so on. There was never a satisfying end-point. A cycle of rumination, he reported, would take well over an hour.

2

Relationship to other disorders

→ Key points

- There is a close association between obsessive–compulsive disorder and depression.

- Some obsessive–compulsive symptoms occur in other psychological disorders, such as social phobias.

- A number of patients with post-traumatic stress disorder have associated symptoms of obsessive–compulsive disorder.

- There is an overlap between eating disorders and obsessive–compulsive disorder in a minority of patients.

- In some cases there is an overlap between obsessive–compulsive disorder and body dysmorphic disorder.

- Morbid jealousy is occasionally associated with obsessive–compulsive disorder.

- There is no relationship between obsessive–compulsive disorders and schizophrenia.

This chapter deals with the relationship between obsessive–compulsive disorder and some other psychological disorders.

Depression

There is a significant relationship between obsessive–compulsive disorder and depression. Roughly three out of four sufferers from obsessive–compulsive disorder have concurrent depression or have experienced clinical depression at some point in their lives. Some people develop obsessions when they become depressed; in such cases the obsessions are essentially secondary to the depression, and generally clear up when the depression lifts. Many obsessive–compulsive patients have a past history of episodes of depression. Other patients become depressed subsequent to the onset of their disorder; it is a depressing problem and can make one feel helpless and hopeless. When depressed, the symptoms of obsessive–compulsive disorder tend to get worse. Research has shown that patients who are severely depressed do not respond well to psychological treatment. In such cases, the depression needs to be treated, usually by medications, before improvement can be expected in the obsessive–compulsive symptoms.

In view of the relationship between the two disorders, a word is necessary about the features of depression. The major features are:

- prolonged, seriously depressed mood;

- loss of energy;

- loss of interest or pleasure in usual activities;

- disturbance of appetite and sleep;

- decline in libido;

- severe slowing or agitation;

- feelings of worthlessness or extreme guilt;

- extensive pessimism;

- suicidal ideas.

Morbid preoccupations

Depressed patients are prone to develop morbid preoccupations (as are people in the general population during phases of low mood). There is some similarity and overlap between obsessions and morbid preoccupations: both consist of intrusive and repetitive ideas. However, preoccupations differ in significant ways from true obsessions in that they centre on realistic current problems or worries, and lack the repugnant or irrational quality of obsessions. They are rarely resisted, and the person usually recognizes them to be reasonable, if exaggerated.

Schizophrenia

The relationship with schizophrenia is more limited. In schizophrenia, stereo-typed behaviour, which may resemble compulsive behaviour, is sometimes evident. It is also known that in the early stages of schizophrenic illness, obsessions and compulsions may appear occasionally, but these are short-lived. Complaints of schizophrenic patients about intrusive thoughts bear a superficial similarity to obsessions, but they generally believe that the thoughts have been inserted into their minds by external forces, human or otherwise. This feature clearly distinguishes them from obsessional thoughts, which the patient recognizes as his own. Other prominent symptoms of schizophrenia, such as delusions and hallucinations, are not encountered in obsessive–compulsive disorder.

Many years ago, some writers and clinicians held the view that obsessive–compulsive disorder and schizophrenia were closely related conditions. The medical literature of the nineteenth century suggested that obsessive–compulsive disorder was a variant of schizophrenia, and it was classified at the time within the spectrum of psychotic disorders. Some authors even took the view that the disorder is a defence against a schizophrenic breakdown. There is no evidence to support this view, and the belief in a connection with schizophrenia is discredited. The chances of an obsessive–compulsive patient developing schizophrenia are no higher than those of any other person.

Phobias

Phobias fall into the category of anxiety disorders, because anxiety is prominent in both of them. Sometimes obsessive–compulsive disorders are confused with phobias, which are excessive and irrational fears. With the important exception of a fear of contamination, patients with obsessive–compulsive disorder do not appear to be particularly prone to develop phobias. The fear of contamination tends to be intense, spreads rapidly, is dominating, and generates widespread avoidance. This fear drives the classical symptom of the disorder—compulsive washing and cleaning.

With this exception, compulsive behaviour of the obsessive–compulsive type is uncommon in phobias. A person who has a phobia usually feels safe in his day-to-day life, if he successfully avoids the object or situation that scares him. Someone with a phobia of elevators, for example, will avoid using elevators and be able to lead an untroubled life, as long as he is not obliged to use an elevator; and someone with a phobia of spiders can lead a normal life, as long as he avoids encounters with spiders. In contrast, an obsessive–compulsive patient cannot escape from his problems as easily; even if he manages to minimize contacts with places/people that trigger his obsessions or compulsive urges, his problems are not contained. Obsessions in particular, frequently intrude at times and places that are not containable. In fact, for many patients the potential 'trigger', an intrusive thought, can emerge any time, anywhere. For example, a woman with obsessive–compulsive disorder may totally avoid knives, scissors, and other sharp objects, which she fears she may use to attack people, but still be tormented by thoughts that she might commit these acts, or be engulfed by self-doubts about whether or not she has already attacked someone. Fears of becoming contaminated by direct physical contact with a dirty/dangerous object (contact contamination) come closest to resembling a phobia, but the related fear of mental contamination, which often arises without any contact, is less like a phobia.

Obsessions and compulsions are more intrusive and more pervasive than phobias, and frequently interfere with daily living.

Eating disorders

Anorexia nervosa

Anorexia nervosa has been described by some writers as a form of obsessive–compulsive disorder. The intense determination to lose weight, and the incessant preoccupation with food, weight, and body size and shape, that these patients display have been given as evidence for this. Anorexics are commonly described as 'obsessed with thinness'. They are certainly preoccupied with their weight, size, and eating. However, anorexia nervosa is a separate disorder, not part of an obsessive–compulsive illness, although there is some relationship between the two, and a proportion of females with obsessive–compulsive disorder do have a past history of anorexia nervosa. A sizeable sub-group of anorexic patients has obsessions and/or compulsions, some of them quite marked; the two disorders coexist. In fact many studies have reported this co-morbidity in a significant minority of anorexic patients. Sometimes, the symptoms of the two disorders influence each other and get intertwined—i.e. certain behaviour assumes significance in both disorders. For example:

An adolescent girl had the compulsive behaviour of running up and down the stairs a certain number of times before every meal. This had all the features of a compulsion, but it could equally be seen as anorexic behaviour, designed to lose weight—and it certainly had that effect. She also had the compulsion to leave a quantity of food on her plate, arranged in a certain way, unconsumed. Her explanation was that she felt compelled to do this. Although she denied that it had anything to do with restricting her eating, the behaviour clearly contributed to maintaining a lower weight.

Patients with both anorexia and obsessive–compulsive problems report that their latter difficulties tend to get worse when they are particularly unhappy with their weight and body size. It is also known that anorexics with obsessive–compulsive symptoms tend to display more severe anorexic disorders than those who do not have such symptoms.

Bulimia nervosa

In bulimia nervosa the patient has recurrent episodes of binge eating, followed by self-induced vomiting and/or laxative abuse. The urge to engage in binge eating is described by some of these patients as having a compulsive quality, although the nature of the behaviour is by no means senseless. As with anorexics, some bulimics also have concomitant obsessive–compulsive problems, some features of which may become closely related to the eating disorder. For example, a young woman with a history of both disorders reported that when she binged on chocolate bars she felt compelled to eat 24 bars at a time, neither more nor fewer, and the binge had to be uninterrupted. If the chocolates got 'contaminated' by the smell of another food, then the bingeing episode had to be restarted.

Post-traumatic stress disorder

Post-traumatic stress disorder is another of the anxiety disorders (see Table 1.1). The psychological effects of severe traumatic experiences are well known, but it is only in recent years that the diagnostic category of post-traumatic stress disorder has been widely recognized. Essentially, this refers to a psychological disorder that some people develop after exposure to a traumatic event (e.g. war, earthquakes and fires, violence, serious motor accidents). The main features are the persistent re-experiencing of the traumatic event—e.g. recurrent intrusive memories, recurrent dreams; avoidance of reminders of the event; and increased arousal, as reflected by sleep difficulties, poor concentration, and so on. Large numbers of war veterans have been treated for this disorder in the USA and elsewhere, and there is an active and still growing interest in this area.

The recurrent, intrusive thoughts and images that occur in this disorder are similar to some of the obsessions experienced by patients with obsessive–compulsive disorder. This is particularly so for the very vivid intrusive images. For example, a former soldier now suffering from post-traumatic stress disorder had the recurrent image of bloated and charred bodies. In addition to very disturbing images, sufferers tend to have intrusive thoughts other than memories of the event (e.g. 'Why did it have to happen to me?', 'Am I really safe now?'). Some also report cognitive compulsions, such as compulsively saying 'No, it wasn't my fault', or compulsively going over the incident, step by step in great detail.

In a small number of patients with this disorder, overt compulsive rituals are found. One, a 46-year-old man who was subjected to a vicious act of violence, developed rituals of repeatedly checking door and window locks. A woman who was seriously sexually assaulted while on holiday began to wash herself compulsively in order to 'become clean'.

It is common for some of the features of obsessive–compulsive disorder and post-traumatic disorder to overlap; but are the two related? There are certainly instances in which a trauma victim develops obsessions and/or compulsions to the degree that one can describe him as suffering from obsessive–compulsive disorder. Numbers of obsessive–compulsive patients have a history of traumatic or disturbing experiences, but the two disorders have distinctive features. The majority of patients with obsessive–compulsive disorder do not have a history of trauma. Similarly, the majority of patients who suffer from post-traumatic stress disorder do not develop full-blown obsessive–compulsive disorder. A small number do, and may have both disorders concurrently. In some, the obsessive–compulsive disorder persists even after the full-blown post-traumatic stress disorder has resolved.

> A married woman in her forties had a horrendous car accident. The car suddenly blew a tyre on a busy road, and when it stopped it was hit by a vehicle coming rather fast from behind. The car went up in flames, and a young child—a friend's son—strapped to a seat, perished. She developed severe post-traumatic stress disorder, with recurrent intrusive images and other symptoms. She began to ask her husband for reassurance, especially about the safety of their own child, and repeatedly checked the child's bedroom at night. She also had the compulsion to visualize the child who died, in bright clothes and smiling. She was guilt-ridden and depressed, and later developed a range of checking and cleaning rituals. When seen 18 months after the accident, she had full-blown obsessive–compulsive disorder.

Gilles de la Tourette syndrome

This condition is characterized by repeated, multiple tics, including vocal tics, which may take the form of swear words or obscenities. These tics are different from true compulsions—they are involuntary, meaningless, and purposeless, unlike compulsions. Nor can they be easily delayed, reshaped, or substituted, again unlike compulsions. The treatment methods that are successful with obsessive–compulsive disorder are of little use with Tourette patients.

It has been reported that some patients with this syndrome also have obsessive–compulsive symptoms, particularly the younger patients. In some studies, first-degree relatives of Tourette patients have also been reported to have a higher incidence of obsessive–compulsive disorder than the general population. Despite these apparent associations, however, the vast majority of patients with obsessive–compulsive disorder do not have Gilles de la Tourette syndrome.

Body dysmorphic disorder

The disorder, which used to be called 'dysmorphophobia', is characterized by excessive concern and preoccupation with imagined defects in bodily appearance. The common complaints are about the face or head (e.g. shape or size of nose, mouth, eyebrows, chin, or jaws). Less commonly, the person may be over-concerned with some other part of the body (such as hands, feet, breasts, or genitals). Asymmetry or lack of proportion can also be a concern. In some cases, cosmetic surgery is sought. The repetitive thoughts in this disorder may resemble obsessions, and the person usually engages in extensive visual checking behaviour, repeatedly checking in the mirror. Reassurance-seeking is very common, and some patients make repeated visits to physicians and surgeons, in search of help and comfort. The patient's conviction that he has a physical abnormality may lead to social avoidance.

Despite the repetitive thoughts and checking, body dysmorphic disorder is distinct from obsessive–compulsive disorder, and is not classified as an anxiety disorder. The delusional self-perceptions that are the hallmark of the dysmorphic disorder are not present in obsessive–compulsive disorders.

Brain damage

Symptoms similar to obsessions and compulsions can result from brain damage caused by injury or neurological disease: the patient may engage in repetitive acts or express repetitive ideas. The appearance of obsessive–compulsive-type symptoms in certain organic conditions (e.g. encephalitis lethargica) has been recognized for many decades. These symptoms are usually accompanied by other signs of brain damage, such as deficits in memory and learning ability. Furthermore, repetitive acts and ideas of these patients are different from obsessions and compulsions in that they lack intellectual content and intentionality, and have a mechanical or primitive quality.

Studies undertaken to investigate the neurological and neuropsychological features of obsessive–compulsive patients have not, up to now, produced consistent or clear-cut results. It is safe to say that there is no evidence of any brain damage in the vast majority of obsessive–compulsive patients.

Obsessional personality

Different views have been expressed on the relationship between obsessive–compulsive disorder and obsessional personality (also called 'compulsive personality' and 'anankastic' personality'). The concept of 'obsessional personality' refers to a group of enduring characteristics in a person, including orderliness, meticulousness, preoccupation with detail, parsimony, obstinacy, neatness, difficulty handling uncertainty, and perfectionism. According to some writers, obsessive–compulsive disorder is only an exaggerated stage or version of an obsessional personality. This is incorrect. Obsessional personality traits are acceptable to the person, seldom cause distress, and are rarely accompanied by a sense of compulsion. They rarely provoke resistance. People seldom seek treatment for an obsessional personality. These personality traits, such as perfectionism, show far greater stability than the manifestations of obsessive–compulsive disorder. Setting and striving to maintain exceedingly high personal standards is remarkably stable; people tend to take pride in their perfectionism, even when it is extreme and a cause for criticism from others (see pp. 60–61 below).

A related view is that obsessional personality traits are a precursor of obsessive–compulsive disorder—i.e. the traits are an early form of the disorder, a sort of risk factor. However, this is not supported by satisfactory evidence. It is true that a proportion of obsessive–compulsive patients do have an obsessional-type personality, but many more with very different personality characteristics also develop the disorder. Conversely, the majority of people with obsessional personalities never develop obsessive–compulsive disorder.

If we were to look for any single personality type that is associated with the disorder, it would perhaps best be described as overly cautious and introverted, rather than obsessional. Even this has to be seen as only a very general observation, as there are numerous exceptions.

Obsessional–compulsive personality disorder

People with obsessional personality features, to a degree that affects their life and functioning, are sometimes described as suffering from an obsessional–compulsive personality disorder, also called 'obsessional personality disorder' or 'compulsive personality disorder'. In these people, the main features are long-standing personality traits, such as excessive rigidity and perfectionism, undue preoccupation with details, indecisiveness, and so on. These features are well established by early adulthood, and are evident in a variety of contexts. In addition, these people tend to show a lack of, or limited ability to express, warm and tender emotions. They do not necessarily have, or develop, true obsessions and compulsions, and rarely feel the need to seek treatment of any kind. Few people with these characteristics attend clinics that deal with psychological problems, and, when they do seek help, it is usually because of depression or difficulties in relationships. This disorder is more common in males than females. Sometimes a patient may display features of this disorder as well as obsessive–compulsive disorder. In such cases a dual diagnosis is given.

Obsessional–compulsive personality disorder is not classified under anxiety disorders. It is essentially a personality disorder, and has little in common with the other anxiety disorders.

Excessive hoarding

As mentioned earlier, nowadays there is uncertainty about whether 'compulsive hoarding' is a particular manifestation of obsessive–compulsive disorders, or is best regarded as a separate problem that is loosely associated with other disorders, such as social anxiety, depression, and obsessive–compulsive disorders. However, there is no uncertainty that excessive hoarding, whether called compulsive or not, can be a serious and intractable problem.

Compulsive hoarding is the intensive collection and retention of large numbers of articles that are useless or of limited value. The affected person takes great care to 'protect' his collections, and experiences emotional resistance to discarding items from the collection. They cling tenaciously to their collections. In extreme forms the compulsive hoarding results in an accumulation of piles of objects that occupy a steadily increasing amount of living space, with the affected person and family members having to navigate their way through mounds of clutter. When a room becomes virtually unusable, it is closed off and the space is turned into an overflow storage area. For example, one patient who engaged in compulsive hoarding filled her double garage to the roof with an enormous collection of articles, none of which she felt able to discard or even sort, and, as a result, the family vehicles had to be parked on the road. Another patient, who lived in a single-bedroom apartment, built up a collection of articles (mainly gifts that she might wish to donate) that gradually occupied the entire bedroom, forcing her to sleep on the couch in the sitting room. Even in this remaining space, she had to thread her way through steadily rising mounds of objects. These objects were placed on the floor and all the furniture, including the bed, with the single exception of one chair, which she used for sitting in when she ate or watched television.

In these extreme cases, the wish to collect and retain unnecessary objects is first an embarrassment and inconvenience, but can evolve into an overwhelming preoccupation that produces distress and an inability to function normally. It can also be hazardous. Common collections include business correspondence (receipts, letters, bank statements, vouchers, and credit card receipts), newspapers, and household goods from toothpaste tubes to dozens of blankets, timetables, and so forth.

Of course, most people will build up a collection of some sort or another, and indeed many people find it difficult to discard some items, even when they are no longer in use; however, the intensity, irrationality, and extent of compulsive hoarding is so obviously out of control as to be unmistakable. The distress arises from the upsetting social consequences of hoarding, plus an anxiety about protecting one's collection, and taking great care to ensure that no one touches or removes or discards items from the hoard. It can distort ordinary functioning because of the severe restrictions that it places on the person's daily life, the physical discomfort, the expense involved, and the inability to tolerate visitors to one's home. Excessive hoarding also provokes unwelcome objections and severe criticism from relatives, neighbours, and health and fire-prevention officials.

The five components of compulsive hoarding are:

◆   the excessive acquisition of very large numbers of unnecessary and often worthless objects/items;

◆   apparently irrational, emotional attachments to the objects;

◆   vigilant protection of the collection;

◆   cluttered living conditions;

◆   an emotional and behavioural inability to discard the objects/items.

It is excessive if it results in an unmanageable clutter, prevents normal daily activities, creates major problems for other people, or if the collection presents fire or health hazards. It tends to be distressing for other people rather than the affected person, except for the upsetting complaints and objections that the hoarder has to endure from other people or authorities.

Accumulating large collections of items can begin early in life but seldom becomes a serious problem until later in life; in contrast, most cases of obsessive–compulsive disorder emerge in adolescence or early adulthood. Hoarders tend to explain their ever-growing collections as necessary in order to ensure that they have the object or item should the need ever arise. They collect large numbers of 'back-ups' and have an inflated fear of the consequences of falling short at some unforeseen time in the future.

Indecisiveness is common in compulsive hoarding. They fret over whether or not to expand their collections of particular items, and, if so, how many additions are necessary. They also have difficulty in deciding which items to retain and which ones to discard. Characteristically, when they attempt to sort and discard unnecessary items, they soon drift into creating new if smaller mounds of objects; they engage in what Dr R. Frost, an American expert who has made extensive studies of this problem, has called 'churning' of the objects, without actually discarding any of them. Patients often experience emotional reactions when they attempt to discard the objects, and these reactions reinforce their fears of what will happen if they lose or throw out an item. A fear of the consequences is particularly acute when the items are hoarded for sentimental reasons, either because of their symbolic value or because of the memories they evoke. In those instances when the person derives an emotional sense of comfort and safety from the collection, their fear of loss is readily understandable. The emotional attachment to worthless, apparently meaningless junk is not easy to understand; presumably, the items have some magical or symbolic value.

Many hoarders describe the comfort they feel when they are with their collected possessions, and prefer to keep their collections in view. They derive a sense of safety. The common belief that compulsive hoarding is the direct result of a period of deprivation, especially in childhood, has not been confirmed by scientific research.

In mild cases, useful reductions in acquisitions can be agreed fairly easily, and, although the process of discarding is more difficult, steady progress can be enhanced by continuing support and supervision.

This is an example of a severe case:

A 55-year-old divorced man was referred for help for his compulsive hoarding. The referral was made as a result of complaints by his neighbours (he lived in a block of flats) who feared the risk of fire. He was reluctant to admit that there was a problem, but came for help as he had little choice. When a psychologist and a nurse visited his home with him, they found it almost impossible to get in. The hallway was cluttered with stacks of paper, mostly old newspapers. All the rooms had hoards of items—old, out-of-date food cans, magazines, pieces of cloth, and lots of odds and ends. Most of the furniture was invisible, and the flat smelt of dust and staleness. There was some sort of 'path' to the bed and to the bathroom. The kitchen was too cluttered for any of the appliances to be accessible. In fact the patient had not used the kitchen for a long time; he had to go out for his meals.

The patient's explanation as to why he kept everything was that he was afraid of throwing away 'important papers' and 'things that might be needed'. It was not clear how he could find anything important or needed in the vast hoards he had.

Excessive hoarding is encountered in a range of other psychological and psychiatric problems and is not associated exclusively with obsessive–compulsive disorder. It occurs among people with certain kinds of eating disorders, mental disorders such as schizophrenia, people who are socially isolated, and among some people who have developed psychiatric problems as a result of brain injuries.

Compulsive hoarding shares some characteristics of other forms of compulsive behaviour, such as repeated checking. However, there are significant differences between compulsive hoarding and other forms of obsessive–compulsive disorder. Compulsive hoarding is seldom accompanied by the internal resistance that is typical of most forms of compulsive behaviour. In the clearly obsessive–compulsive problems, the affected person almost always goes through a period during which he or she attempts to resist and prevent the needlessly repetitive behaviour, such as cleaning or checking over and over again. In cases of compulsive hoarding, however, the person generally feels that the collection and retention of these objects is desirable, justifiable, and even necessary, but simply has got out of hand. Few of them feel that their collecting is a psychological problem, and see no need for treatment. They are brought to the attention of health services at the prompting of relatives, neighbours, or others. If necessary, they reluctantly agree to participate in treatment but are inclined to 'negotiate' rather than actively discard their collections. They are more willing to refrain from adding too many new items.

As far as treatment is concerned, neither the medications nor the cognitive behaviour therapy methods that are effective in treating obsessive–compulsive disorders, are effective in managing compulsive hoarding. Research is being conducted but at present there is no specific treatment beyond supportive therapy. Attempts are made to encourage and assist the person to stop acquiring new items. Discarding the objects can be emotionally difficult, however, and the process tends to be slow and gradual. An obstacle to treatment is that many or most people who engage in excessive hoarding do not see it as a psychological problem, and rarely seek treatment. They are not motivated to change. When treatment is attempted, it usually is at the behest of relatives, neighbours, health authorities, or fire departments.

Morbid jealousy

Morbid jealousy is sometimes taken for an obsessive–compulsive disorder because the affected person typically engages in a form of compulsive behaviour, predominantly checking to determine whether his partner is completely faithful, trustworthy, and has a completely acceptable moral history. The driving force is a fixed belief that the partner might be disloyal and untrustworthy. The belief is tenacious and relatively unaffected by evidence, even when the affected person recognizes in a calm state that his suspicions are irrational, shameful, and, at times, absurd. The repeated urges to check on the partner's trustworthiness, and even morality, frequently reach irresistible levels. The morbid jealousy is then manifested in attempts to collect information about the distrusted partner by direct or indirect means. Barely disguised interrogations are typical, and the search for clues spreads widely.

The jealousy and distrust are fixated on one person at a time, generally the current partner, and usually have a sexual component. The concept of morbid jealousy does not include envy of other peoples' possessions, status, or successes. When the affected person transfers his interest and affection to a new partner, the distrust soon follows; it is a 'transferable fixation'. The distrust of the former partner tends to fade and even disappear.

A less common form of morbid jealousy is the drive to learn everything possible, or not possible, about any relationships or even friendships that one's partner had from adolescence onwards. The affected person repeatedly has intense urges to question his partner about all of the details, and returns time and time again to the same subject. In a sense, it is a type of inverse scrupulosity (see p. 61); in morbid jealousy, the person is repeatedly seeking 'the entire truth', rather than repeatedly 'confessing the entire truth' about his own faults and misdemeanours. These powerful urges to find out all of the details of the partner's past end when the relationship ends; the morbid curiosity shifts to a new partner.

The common features in morbid jealousy and obsessive–compulsive disorder are compulsive urges and accompanying behaviour, but the underlying problem in morbid jealousy is an irrational, circumscribed, fixated conviction that one's partner might be disloyal and untrustworthy.

3

Obsessive–compulsive patients

> **Key points**
>
> ◆ The most common forms of obsessive–compulsive disorder are compulsive cleaning and/or compulsive checking, and obsessions.
>
> ◆ The patient feels compelled to carry out repetitive activities over and over again, despite recognition that the behaviour is irrational.
>
> ◆ These compulsions are purposeful, meaningful, and deliberate.
>
> ◆ In most instances they are carried out in an attempt to avert or reduce a sense of danger.
>
> ◆ Obsessions are recurrent unwanted, distressing, often repugnant intrusive thoughts (or images, or impulses).
>
> ◆ In many cases, the patient is afflicted by obsessions and compulsions.
>
> ◆ Many patients attempt to control or limit their symptoms by engaging in strenuous avoidance of particular places, people, or activities.

There are several common forms of obsessive–compulsive disorder. Most patients have more than one problem, but usually there are one or two that are predominant at a given time. When seeking help, patients with obsessive–compulsive disorders tend to be extremely anxious, depressed, frustrated, and in considerable distress. Those with a severe disorder may even be desperate.

It is customary to rank the seriousness of the person's obsessive–compulsive disorder into mild, moderate, or severe.

This broad classification is based on:

◆ The amount of distress the person is experiencing.

◆ The extent to which it interferes with normal functioning.

◆ The degree to which the disorder absorbs the person's mental and physical energy.

◆ Responsiveness to treatment.

◆ The extent to which the person has been reduced to an obsessional life-style, in which the disorder dominates their life.

The ranking of severity provides a basis for recommending the type and intensity of treatment, and also for providing advice about management and the likely course of the disorder.

Main clinical types

Those with:

◆ washing/cleaning compulsions as the major problem;

◆ checking compulsions as the major problem;

◆ other forms of compulsion as the major problem;

◆ obsessions unaccompanied by observable compulsive behaviour;

◆ primary obsessional slowness.

For some time excessive hoarding was included as a form of obsessive–compulsive disorder, but nowadays there is uncertainty about whether or not hoarding should be regarded as a separate problem (see p. 35 above).

The two most common forms of obsessive–compulsive disorder are compulsive washing/cleaning and compulsive checking.

Washers/cleaners

Typically, the patient complains about, and displays a fear of, being contaminated by dirt or germs, or potentially dangerous substances such as chemicals. Substances that are generally feared include bodily products (e.g. blood, seminal fluids, urine, faeces), germs/viruses (especially HIV and SARS), and chemicals such as cleaning products, herbicides, and pesticides. Places that are feared and avoided include public toilets, restaurants, public transport, rough areas of town, and hospitals. In many instances, it is other people who are regarded as a source of contamination. In a minority of cases the person dreads contact with dirty or disgusting objects, people, or places, but is not particularly concerned about contamination. Compulsive cleaning is aimed at protecting oneself and others from the spread of germs or other perceived dangers and/or dirt.

If the patient has been unable to avoid coming into contact with a possible source of contamination, he feels anxious and extremely uncomfortable. These unpleasant feelings quickly generate a compulsive urge to remove the contaminant as quickly and fully as possible. The site of the contamination is generally focused on the hands, because most contacts with the outside world involve our hands. Hence the compulsive urge to remove the contamination is usually directed at washing one's hands. When the person feels extensively contaminated, the urges to wash are correspondingly broader. The washing and cleaning is carried out meticulously. In mild cases, the urges are not powerful and the person manages to contain the washing compulsions by developing cleaning habits that are effective, convenient, and unobtrusive. In severe cases, however, the fear of contamination and the urges can be so overwhelming as to interfere with normal living. Affected people engage in intensive, prolonged washing and wide avoidance. Some patients wash their hands over a hundred times a day, use many bottles of disinfectants/detergents, hundreds of sheets of toilet papers, bathe or shower for several hours a day, and repeatedly wash and wipe table tops, chairs, and floors. The fear of contamination and the ensuing washing and cleaning dominate the person's life.

The avoidance can be extensive. The patient may avoid objects that others have touched, such as door knobs and public telephones; he probably refrains from using public toilets, and avoids sitting on chairs that others sat on, or—if he did—would first cover it with a towel or cloth or sit on the edge. In severe cases, the entire world, except a small area in the home, is avoided. One woman was so concerned about dirt and germs that she felt free only in her bedroom and the bathroom, which she did not allow anyone else to enter. When she went out she wore a large coat and gloves, which she immediately washed upon returning. All items brought into the bedroom had to be cleaned or washed first. Another patient felt some safety only when sitting in her exclusive chair at home; she disinfected her chair daily (see below). Another patient reported that the entire city in which she lived had became so contaminated that she had felt compelled to move to a distant city. She never again went anywhere near the contaminated city, and avoided as best she could anyone who visited it.

The following are illustrations of mild cases:

> A student who had an excessive fear of developing AIDS as a result of contact with a range of places, people, or objects sought treatment because of a spreading feeling that his clothes were becoming contaminated. Initially he was upset when he inadvertently walked close to a discarded condom in a rough part of the city. Over the next few days his fear of having contracted AIDS escalated and he laundered all of the clothes that he had been wearing during the incident. He was particularly sensitized to his shoes and wrapped them in several layers of plastic before depositing them on a high shelf in the storeroom. He was aware that his fears of AIDS were exaggerated and unrealistic.
>
> Following the incident, he began to wash his hands more frequently and avoided various places that were associated with AIDS. However, he continued to function normally in most circumstances and progressed well in his studies. After five sessions of exposure treatment, the fear of contamination receded and he was able to resume wearing his shoes and other affected clothing.

> A man became increasingly worried and then frightened by the possibility that he might inadvertently contaminate food that he was preparing in the kitchen. He attempted to deal with the problem by adopting extremely strict cleaning practices and by washing his hands up to 40 times per day. He was troubled by these changes and tried very hard to control them, but without success. His social and other activities were unaffected. After a course of cognitive behaviour therapy, the fear and associated cleaning compulsions were brought under control.

These are illustrations of severe cases, in which the person's life has become dominated by the obsessive–compulsive disorder:

> A woman had obsessions about dirt, and related compulsions. Her main concern was about excrement, both human and animal. She would wash extensively after returning from a walk, even if she did not actually see, let alone step on, dirt. This was because she felt that dog dirt is spread all over the roads and pavements by rain and wind. She would leave her

shoes outside the door and change into a different pair before entering the house. She totally avoided public toilets. As the problem got worse, she began to avoid going anywhere near manholes because they indicated the presence of sewers with human excreta underneath. She would avoid parts of roads in her area where she knew there were manholes. By the time she came for help, she had almost stopped going out, left her job, and had begun to spend much of her time in bed. She also began to demand that her parents, with whom she lived, stop going out, as they would bring dirt into the house when they returned, and to insist that they left their shoes outside and washed their hands and feet when they returned from an outing. She was in considerable distress and unable to function normally.

A married woman in her mid-thirties developed a severe and pervasive fear of contracting cancer through contact with any person who had the disease, or places associated with cancer. She recognized that her fear was scientifically groundless but, despite this, it was intense. In order to reduce the chances of contracting cancer, she spent hours each day washing, cleaning, and disinfecting herself and her clothes. As she felt unsafe outside her home, she refrained from leaving it except for the most urgent reasons. She felt more secure in one room of the house, and on one chair in particular, which she disinfected every day. Her hands were red, swollen, and abraded from excessive washing. She was trapped by her obsessive–compulsive disorder, which dictated her every move and left her disabled.

The hands of many compulsive hand-washers show clear signs of excessive washing. The repeated washing tends to dry the natural oils in the skin and frequently causes marked dryness, especially in the areas between the fingers.

Fear of dirt and germs—a patient's account

This is a patient's own account of her washing and cleaning compulsions. She was in her fifties, and lived on her own in an apartment:

 ## Patient perspective

'I cannot touch anything that I think is dirty. It is mainly the toilet, but then when you come out of the toilet, you bring the dirt and the germs out into other parts of the house. I always wash my hands many times before I leave the toilet. I keep my shoes and slippers outside the door of the toilet, so I can step into them as I come out. No, I would never use a public toilet, never. I nearly died when once a young man who came in to fix something used my toilet. He just came out and went on touching things, walking about the place, as if everything was fine! I couldn't tell him to stop, but it was so *awful*. I cleaned and cleaned all over the house after he left. I used disinfectant on the things he touched, even the things he went near. I don't like people coming into my home, not even friends, any more. My bedroom I somehow keep clean. Every other part of the house is really dirty, however much I clean. The towels I have in the toilet I wash separately, never with my other things. When I feel I am dirty I wash and wash, with lots of soap, and with Dettol and whatnot. The whole house smells of disinfectant. I feel fine for a while when I have washed but, when I go to the toilet again, even to pick up something or to open the window, it starts all over again. I don't think I can allow myself to be touched by anyone. I keep my gloves on when I am in shops or on the bus. All the clothes I wear for outside, I never bring into the bedroom without first washing them. If the bedroom also got dirty then I would be finished. Where could I go? That is the only clean place which I have.'

As in the previous case, this patient was trapped and unable to function normally.

The germ war of Howard Hughes

It is well known that the late American millionaire Howard Hughes (1905–76) had severe fears of contamination, and associated compulsions and avoidance behaviour, particularly in the later years of his life. Among other problems, he developed complicated rituals for handling objects. For example, before handing a spoon to Hughes, his attendants were required to wrap the handle in tissue paper and seal it with cellophane tape. A second piece of tissue paper was then wrapped over the first protective wrapping. On receiving the spoon, Hughes would use it with the handle still covered. He gave even more detailed instructions for many other activities, all related to his intense fear of germs and contamination, and his staff had to adhere to these instructions very strictly. Typical of these were his instructions on how to remove his hearing-aid cord from the bathroom cabinet. First, 6–8 Kleenex tissues had to be used for touching the door knob to open the bathroom door. Then the taps were to be opened, using the same tissues, to obtain warm water. Next, 6–8 Kleenex tissues were to be used to open the cabinet that contained the soap, and an unused bar of soap taken. The hands were then to be washed thoroughly, making sure that they did not touch the taps or the sides of the bowl. Next, 15–20 new Kleenex tissues had to be used to turn off the taps. Now the door of the cabinet that contained the hearing-aid cord was to be opened, using at least 15 Kleenexes. Nothing inside the cabinet was to be touched in any way, except the sealed envelope that contained the cord. This was to be removed with both hands, using at least 15 Kleenexes for each hand. Only the centres of the tissues were to be allowed to come into contact with the envelope.

On those occasions when his staff had to touch him in order to wake him up, Hughes's instructions were that the chosen person should pinch his toes with eight thicknesses of Kleenex tissues, applying progressively greater pressure until he woke up.

He was afflicted by a despairingly severe form of obsessive–compulsive disorder, which incidentally illustrates how it is possible for people to carry out some of the patient's compulsions when requested to do so. Parents of children with severe obsessive–compulsive disorders often are drawn into carrying out 'protective' compulsive cleaning by the affected child. Compulsive behaviour is not mere meaningless repetition but is purposeful and deliberate.

Mental contamination

In addition to the familiar type of contamination that is evoked by contact with dangerous/dirty items or situations, there is a less obvious type that can have widespread consequences. Mental contamination can arise from an experience of psychological violation, physical or emotional. Common precipitants include betrayal, humiliation, degradation, being made to feel worthless, and also physical violations such as beatings and sexual assaults.

The feelings of mental contamination share some qualities with contact contamination but have some distinctive features. Feelings of mental contamination can be evoked by mental events such as images, memories, severely critical remarks, and long-distance conversations—even in the absence of any physical contact with a dangerous/dirty object. The affected person generally has some difficulty in locating the source and the site of the contamination because the feelings of pollution seem to be internal rather than the familiar feelings of contamination caused by contact, which are mostly located on the hands. Partly because these feelings involve internal dirtiness and are so unfamiliar, the usual resorting to vigorous washing tends to be ineffective. 'No matter how many times I wash my hands, they still feel dirty.' If the feelings of dirtiness are internal, washing one's hands cannot easily remove them. 'I have to shower over and over again, as many as 10 times, because one or two showers won't do it; I feel as dirty as when I began.'

Many victims of sexual assault report feelings of extreme dirtiness but it is not only dirtiness of the familiar kind. They tend to experience a strong sensation of internal dirtiness that has emotional overtones. 'Things look clean but they feel dirty, shameful. Even after I have taken a shower my friends can tell that I am dirty. It is gross. I feel sullied.' This form of internal dirtiness, a sense of mental pollution, can arise even without physical contact with a dirty object or situation. It is commonly associated with a number of disturbing emotions, among which feelings of shame, disgust, and embarrassment are prominent. Mental pollution is not easily responsive to washing or cleaning. A patient described how she would take five, six, or seven showers in rapid succession in her vain attempts to eliminate the sense of internal dirtiness. Frequent showering had so damaged the wooden floor in her bathroom that it had to be entirely replaced. When asked why one shower was not sufficient, she explained that at best it would give her some marginal relief and, as she was left with a strong sense of dirtiness, she felt compelled to repeat the shower, over and over again. Her feelings of contamination developed after a serious family quarrel in which she had been degraded and subsequently ostracized. Intense feelings of contamination were repeatedly provoked by recurring images and memories of her humiliation.

A distinctive feature of mental contamination is that the source is almost always human, unlike the familiar contamination that is caused by physical contact with dangerous/dirty inanimate items. Take the case of betrayal, which can produce strong and lasting feelings of mental contamination. After returning from a business trip, a man discovered that during his absence, his live-in fiancée had secretly invited an ex-boyfriend to spend several days with her in the flat. She initially denied that the boyfriend had been with her and that they had resumed a sexual relationship. When she divulged to him what had taken place during his absence, the relationship between them was terminated and she moved out. Shortly after these events the affected man began to develop strong feelings of contamination and washed himself repeatedly. He was unable to touch any of his fiancée's few remaining possessions and the feelings of contamination then spread to his own clothing, particularly to those items that had some association with his fiancée. He had many items of his clothing laundered, but that proved to be minimally effective and he stopped wearing them for fear of contamination.

The unresponsiveness to ordinary washing is characteristic of feelings of mental pollution and other forms of mental contamination. Feelings of mental contamination and pollution can be induced by a physical contact, which the affected person finds disgusting, or even by information, and can also be revived by memories or images even in the absence of any physical contacts. The potential for re-contamination is almost always present. Given these qualities, it is not surprising that feelings of mental contamination tend to be so persistent. In order to overcome obsessive–compulsive disorder in patients with a dominant sense of mental contamination, it is necessary to deal with this component of the disorder.

Checkers

People with checking compulsions form the second largest clinical group of obsessive–compulsive patients. Males and females are found in roughly equal numbers in this group. Affected people repeatedly check things such as gas taps, ovens, electrical appliances and switches, door locks, windows, cupboards, drawers, cabinets, or files. The checking is associated with doubting and indecision. 'Did I switch off the gas?', 'I may have left the oven on', 'I might have left the door unlocked', and so on. These doubts produce such anxiety and distress that they drive compulsive urges to check and recheck. The actions are repeated many times (not infrequently a fixed number of times) and, even then, some patients may continue to feel uneasy and unhappy. Checking once is rarely sufficient. The checking takes time and it can be embarrassing and even disabling. One woman was not able to park her car and leave it until she had checked all the switches, radio, aerial, and all doors and windows several times. She would walk around the car, looking and checking before leaving it. Some patients drive back home when they are half-way to work in order to check their gas taps, light switches, and door locks.

Paradoxically, checking causes more checking: the larger the number of checks carried out, the greater the person's uncertainty. They find it increasingly difficult to remember how many times they have checked, and even more difficult to remember if they have checked adequately. The uncertainty promotes urges to re-check, and, in time, the affected person begins to lose confidence in his memory, and may even come to believe that he has had a significant and permanent loss of memory. Actually, this is rare—it is a loss of confidence in one's memory and is specific to tasks or situations in which they feel a strong urge to check for safety. If the affected person observes someone else doing the checking, his memory of the checking behaviour is accurate—providing the other person is fully responsible for the checking. In similar fashion, repeated checking can lead to a loss of confidence in one's ability to attend satisfactorily: 'I can't seem to concentrate properly any more and therefore have to check and re-check. Did I do it correctly?'.

Most checkers strive to make sure that they have excluded any chance of harm coming to themselves or others. Their fear is that disasters will occur if they do not check satisfactorily. Compulsive checking is strongly associated with the fear of being responsible for harm coming to other people or to oneself. A highly inflated sense of responsibility is the underlying problem in most cases of compulsive checking. The two other factors that play a significant part in compulsive checking are gross over-estimations of the probability of a disaster occurring, accompanied by a gross over-estimation of the seriousness of the feared disaster.

An experienced pharmacist was constantly tormented by the probability that he would make an error in preparing a prescription, and that it might lead to a fatality. Each workday he feared that he was likely to make such an error and, consequently, checked each prescription many times over, often seeking reassurance from his colleagues. On a simple scale of probabilities, he estimated that there was a 100% likelihood that he would make a major error within the next 5 days. On the same scale, he estimated that the probability of equally experienced colleagues making a major error in the next 5 days was 000.1%. He felt that errors were most likely to occur when he had overall responsibility; when he was under direct supervision and had less responsibility, he anticipated fewer errors. This is a common biased belief in compulsive checking—'it will happen *because* I am responsible'.

We then calculated that he had prepared approximately 10 000 prescriptions since he qualified. He had made two minor clerical errors. The tenacity of the grossly inflated estimates of making serious mistakes is a common problem in therapy.

An experienced plumber had to check and re-check every plumbing job he had done, however small. If he did not do this, he felt that the pipes would burst and the building would be flooded. He sometimes invented excuses to return to houses where he had done a job, in order to repeat his checking. In some cases, the disasters feared were remote, and not in any way connected to the behaviour—such as air crashes involving relatives, or even earthquakes.

While many checkers are excessively worried about ensuring the safety of doors and gas taps, some of them have less easily understood concerns.

A patient may check every chair for pins or sharp objects, or for pieces of glass. For example, one man compulsively checked every garbage bag that he walked past to make sure that it contained just rubbish, and not a corpse. Another man repeatedly drove back along the way he had just gone, to check if he had knocked down a pedestrian or an animal. Retracing one's path or journey is a relatively common form of compulsive checking.

A man in his late twenties was referred with extensive checking behaviour. He felt compelled to check that 'everything was right', so he would go back over everything he did. The most serious doubts he had were about doors, widows, and gas taps, which he checked several times before leaving the house in the morning and before retiring to bed at night. He also checked anything that he wrote several times, which delayed his work considerably. He could not put anything in an envelope or a file, drawer, or cabinet without repeatedly checking that he had written exactly the right thing. He often ripped opened sealed envelopes to re-read what he had written. He also checked the dates of newspapers: while reading a newspaper, he would check repeatedly that it was that day's; even if had just been delivered to him. Some of his checking, he felt, was necessary to avoid fires, the house being burgled, the bathroom getting flooded, and so on. For the rest, he had only a vague notion that it was necessary to avoid some unspecified calamity. At the time that he came for help, he was seriously affected by the problem; nothing could be left unchecked, and his work was becoming impossible.

The patients in all of these examples had an exaggerated sense of responsibility and felt that it was incumbent upon them to prevent errors of disasters from taking place. To this end, they felt compelled to carry out their checking rituals.

When the feeling of responsibility of such patients is transferred or suspended, the compulsive checking tends to decline or even stop altogether. So, for example, a person who feels compelled to carry out repeated checks of the light switches, gas taps, and so on in his own house is free of these compulsions when visiting the houses of other people. If seriously affected people are admitted to hospital for in-patient treatment, they typically show little or no checking behaviour in the first few days. As they settle in, however, they begin to feel responsible for the security of the ward and their checking re-emerges.

Mild cases of compulsive checking generally respond well to psychological treatment:

> The assistant manager of a large sporting-goods shop dreaded those few occasions on which he was the last person to leave, and was responsible for securing the building. He was convinced that a fire or robbery would occur on these occasions and rated the probability at 80%. Consequently, he checked repeatedly and ritualistically, for as long as 2 hours. If the patient was present when the manager closed up at the end of the day, he rated the probability of a disaster as less than 1%. Both the probability and seriousness of a disaster were extremely inflated whenever he felt responsible. He also feared that when driving he might inadvertently and unknowingly harm a pedestrian, and as result repeatedly checked his rear view mirror. Not infrequently he felt compelled to re-trace his journey in order to allay he fear that he might have harmed someone. He responded well to a short course of cognitive behaviour therapy.

> An athletic runner sought assistance because she feared that she might harm, even kill, a stranger while she was running on forest paths that were somewhat obscured. As in the previous case, she often felt compelled to re-trace her path in order to confirm that she had not left someone injured or killed. She, too, responded well to a short course of cognitive behaviour therapy.

Both of these people had high personal standards and an inflated sense of responsibility. Characteristically, they volunteered for charitable enterprises, and were regarded in their families as being exceptionally sympathetic and dependable.

Those with other types of observable compulsions

There are some patients whose main problem consists of compulsions that do not fall into the above categories. There is no preponderance of either males or females in this heterogeneous group. Common examples are associated with strong feelings about particular numbers, letters, or even colours that are perceived to be 'unsafe', and therefore must be avoided. This form resembles intense superstitions, except that the thoughts about the numbers and so forth are extreme, intrusive, personal, and always negative. One patient spent a lot of mental effort trying to avoid using his three 'unsafe' letters and evolved a range of tricks to substitute words that did not contain the dreaded letters. The origin of his unsafe feelings was tracked to a traumatic experience of abandonment, and that particular word became sensitized. Some patients feel compelled to repeat certain behaviour, such as washing, a rigidly determined number of times, say washing each finger four times before moving on to the next finger. One woman had the compulsion to go back into the bathroom three times after a bath or wash, before she could go on to other things. Some have to do things in a certain way—e.g. a strict sequence has to be followed in preparing a meal or setting the table. Each step has a predetermined place in the sequence of behaviour. Some have touching compulsions—e.g. touching corners of a room, touching with one hand what has been touched with the other, and ensuring equal contact time for each hand. Some of the behaviour appears bizarre to others, and patients may try to conceal the compulsive behaviour.

The reason that many of patients give for doing these things is usually the same as that given by checkers: if they do not do it, serious harm will come to themselves or to a loved one. In some instances, feared disaster is very specific, but in others it is a vague feeling of harm or danger.

Carried to extremes, even list-making can become compulsive. Every day the patient makes lengthy lists of things to do, items to buy, people to telephone, and so on—well beyond the bounds of reason. One woman had to make a detailed list each morning of every single thing that she had to do during the day, including such routine activities as having breakfast, going to the toilet, putting on shoes. When each behaviour was completed, it was crossed off the list. Items not on the list could not be performed. This behaviour was so time-consuming that she was late for everything. When her mother once took away her notebook, she began to write on the palms of her hands.

Other overt compulsions include completing things, arranging things in symmetrical order or in some other regular way, straightening things, looking at things in a certain way, or looking at particular things, colours, and so on. One patient was unable to leave her room until a large array of her belongings was placed in their exact positions. No one was allowed to enter her room without her and, even then, they were obliged to avoid moving any of the items. Another variant centres on the serious discomfort arising when interrupted by unwanted intrusions. For example, while making tea, if one hears the word 'death' or 'murder' on the radio, or happens to see a 'dirty' object like a waste bin, interruptions may require that the whole operation is started afresh. This is repeated until a 'clear run' is achieved. Sometimes the person feels compelled to achieve a 'clear head' even before starting to arrange, straighten, or settle objects. The type of event that can disrupt a behaviour and necessitate a repetition is usually something to do with dirt, danger, or illness; but it can also be something of a personal relevance (such as hearing the name of a loved one) or a senseless triviality (e.g. hearing words beginning with 'z'). Patients who are troubled by intrusive blasphemous obsessions tend to encounter difficulties in praying. If a blasphemous image or thought intrudes when the person is praying, it is necessary to begin all over again because the intrusion has discoloured the prayer.

A patient's account of her day

A 20-year-old woman was in hospital for another problem at the time that she wrote this account of a day as an in-patient. As can be seen, 'number rituals' dominated her life. Her problems had started when she was a child.

 Patient's perspective

During the course of the night, I get in and out of the bed four times.

7 a.m. I get out of bed for the fourth time, put my contact lenses in and take them out four times, then make my bed, folding each corner four times, straightening the blankets and tucking them in four times, arranging the pillows four times, pulling the bed away from the wall and pushing it back in place four times, folding and unfolding the extra blankets four times, straightening the top cover four times, and drawing the curtains back and forth four times. I go to the toilet, put the lid of the toilet down and lift it up again four times, wash my hands four times, and go to the lounge counting my steps in fours in my head. I look at each corner of the room four times, counting the chairs in the room four times, and go back to the dormitory counting four times. I then pick up my washbag and put it down four times, go to the washroom counting in fours, pull the curtain back and forth four times, wash each part of my body four times, clean my contact lenses four times, brush my teeth and hair four times, and go back to the dormitory counting in fours.

8 a.m. Breakfast—I pull my chair in at the table four times, recite in my head four different prayers four times, use the pepper four times, putting it on four different places on my plate, put my knife and fork down four times during the meal, chew the food four times or in multiples of four, and use four teaspoons of coffee, stirring it four times. I get up from the table and go to the lounge counting in fours, get up and sit down four times, say four different prayers four times, touch each corner of the chair four times. I now shower—I step in and out of the shower four times, switch the water on and off four times, wash each part of my body four times, shampoo my hair four times, rinse my hair and flannel four times, dry each part of my body four times, put my nightdress on and take it off four times. After cleaning out each drawer of my bedside locker four times, I fold up the clothes in my wardrobe four times, change the water in the flower vase four times, dry my hair with the hair-dryer while counting in fours, put my washing into the washing machine and take it out four times, switch the machine on and off four times, and tidy the toiletries on my locker while counting in fours, picking each item up and putting it down four times. I go to the telephone counting in fours, pick up the receiver and put it down four times before dialling, look at the dial four times, and put the receiver down and pick it up four times at the end of the conversation. After going back to the washroom counting in fours, I pull the curtains back and forth four times, go to the toilet, put down the lid and lift it up four times, wash my hands and clean my contact lenses four times, blow my nose four times, and recite in my head four different prayers four times.

Noon Lunch—I pull my chair in at the table four times, look at each person at the table four times before each course, cut each piece of food into four pieces or multiples of four, chew each piece of food four times, and swallow, counting in fours. I wipe my hands on my flannel four times, then go to the lounge counting my steps in fours, sit down and stand up four times, take my slippers off and put them back on four times, touch each corner of the chair four times, look at each corner of the room four times, look at each person in the room four times.

6 p.m. Supper—I pull my chair in at the table four times, look at each person at the table four times, and use the pepper four times.

10 p.m. I queue up for medication and count each person in the queue four times, go through to the washroom counting my steps in fours, wash each part of my body four times, brush my teeth four times, blow my nose four times, and go to the toilet, putting the lid down and lifting it up four times, then washing my hands four times. I go back to the dormitory counting my steps in fours, pull back the bedcovers four times, take out my contact lenses and put them back in four times, get in and out of bed four times, hang up my dressing gown four times, draw the curtains four times, take off my slippers and put them back on four times, get in and out of bed again four times, say four different prayers four times, touch each corner of the pillow four times, and turn over in bed four times.

Those with obsessions unaccompanied by observable compulsions

There are patients whose obsessive–compulsive disorder is characterized chiefly by mental events, with no overt compulsions. As noted earlier, obsessions can be thoughts, images, impulses, or combinations of these (see Table 1.3). The majority of obsessions consist of unwanted, unacceptable, and even repugnant intrusions, and the content is blasphemous and/or aggressive and/or unacceptable sexual thoughts. Patients tend to interpret these objectionable intrusions as possibly signifying that they are 'mad, bad, or dangerous'. The intrusions are recurrent and disturbing, and provoke feelings of guilt, anxiety, and self-doubt.

In some patients, the obsessions are followed by covert compulsions, or mental rituals, which are comparable with observable behavioural compulsions in that they result from a strong compulsive urge and usually have the effect of bringing about some temporary relief. Such mental compulsive rituals include silent counting, uttering prayers or certain words and phrases silently, or conjuring up certain visual images. The mental compulsions are used as a means of cancelling or neutralizing the obsession, and/or preventing the harm associated with it.

> A married woman referred herself for help with what she described as 'unwanted ideas', which were about the possibility of her going mad. She had an aunt with a mental illness who spent most of her life in a large mental hospital. For some time, our patient had been assailed by the obsessions 'Am I going mad?', 'Will I end up insane?', 'Will I be locked up?', and so on. Sometimes, she also experienced visual images of herself locked up in a hospital cell. The thoughts, and the images to a lesser extent, made her extremely anxious and sometimes quite depressed. She reported that the thoughts came 'at least a hundred times a day'. Her husband, to whom she turned for reassurance, somehow did not understand how distressed she was by these, and tended to laugh them off, which made her feel even more helpless. She had no compulsive rituals, either overt or covert.

The following is an example of obsessions with associated mental compulsive behaviour:

> A devout man was so deeply troubled by recurrent sexual images of the Virgin Mary that he was unable to continue attending church. He avoided all pictures and reminders of her and prayed for forgiveness for the sin of blasphemy. Whenever an image of the Virgin intruded, he strained to replace it with an image of a peaceful countryside scene, and repeatedly uttered a neutralizing prayer.

This is an example of a mental compulsive behaviour, with no associated obsession:

> A young man had the unwanted compulsion of silently repeating everything other people said in conversation. This meant that he had to be very alert, as he could not afford to miss a single word. The effect of this was that often he could not keep up with conversations, as his own contributions were necessarily limited. At the time he came for help, the compulsion had also spread to what he heard on the radio and television; he often missed the general meaning of what was being said because he was so busy mechanically repeating the words that were being uttered.

Mental compulsions—a patient's account

The following is an account of an elaborate mental compulsive ritual, as described by a patient. The man, in his late thirties, reported having had this problem for over a year. He also had some other obsessive–compulsive problems, but they were relatively minor.

 Patient perspective

The thought is that something awful is going to happen, not to me but to my family. It happens dozens of times a day—on some days over 50 times. It can happen at any time, but more when I am on my own. Sometimes it is an accident, sometimes a certain illness, sometimes even death; it is not always clear which. What is clear is that something terrible is going to happen. It comes into my mind sharply, all of a sudden, and when it comes I cannot get rid of it. Whatever I might be doing at the time (say, reading a book) has to stop. The thought dominates everything else. It makes me quite anxious, and very tense. I know that it is irrational to worry about my family simply because of a silly thought but, when the thought comes, I do worry. I then have to put it right somehow: I have to cancel out the thought. I don't remember how it began, but what I do now when I get this thought is to imagine certain things. It is a very fixed sequence. I have to visualize pictures of my children, my wife, my parents—who are both dead now—then pictures of the Virgin Mary and Jesus Christ, and then pictures of two other people whom I happen to know. They have to come in that order, and always the picture of my daughter Jean has to be imagined before the picture of my son Tom. When I imagine pictures of the Virgin Mary and Jesus Christ, they have to have little gold-yellow lights around them. I don't always get these images easily; in fact, it is often quite a struggle. If it goes wrong or if I am disturbed when I am visualizing these pictures, I have to start again.

Most of all, even when I have imagined the whole sequence completely, if I then see something dirty, like shoes or a waste bin, straight afterwards, then this makes the whole thing worthless, so I have to start again. When it is done without any such mishap, I feel greatly relieved. The tension and the uneasiness all go, and I can get back to whatever I was doing. I somehow feel that I have ensured that the family will be safe, that the disaster that I feared will now not happen. Of course, this is not rational or logical, but that is how I feel at the time.

Getting 'a clear run'

Patients who suffer from persistently intrusive, repugnant thoughts sometimes find that actions that are carried out when their nasty thoughts or images are present have to be repeated again and again. In order to gain relief, they find that they have first to achieve a neutral thought or image, and then carry out the action. For example, a 17-year-old student who repeatedly brushed her hair, taking up to 2 hours on occasions, explained that, in order to feel 'satisfied' with her hair, she had to brush it when she had a neutral or good thought in mind. If she experienced one of her objectionable, obscene, intrusive thoughts while brushing her hair, the entire action was spoilt and she had to begin again. On bad days, when the thoughts were especially persistent, she ended up spending long and frustrating periods trying to 'get her hair right'. As mentioned earlier, if prayers become discoloured by objectionable intrusive images or thoughts, the person is likely to try clearing his mind before re-starting the prayer.

Primary obsessional slowness

There are a small number of patients, mostly male, whose problem is best described as 'primary obsessional slowness'. This condition was first identified about 40 years ago, and cases have been reported from several countries. Most obsessive–compulsive patients are slow as a result of their repetitive behaviour, but, in this group, slowness is the primary problem; it is not secondary to any ritualistic behaviour. The patient may take half an hour to brush his teeth, an hour to shave, four hours to bathe, and so on. The behaviour is extremely meticulous and precise. Each task has to be done in a self-prescribed ritualistic manner, in the correct sequence, and in an unchanging manner from day to day. The actions most affected in this way are self-care behaviour and other simple tasks of daily living, although, in a minority, behaviour at work is also affected. In practice, however, such extreme slowness in self-care behaviour makes a working life virtually impossible.

In one severe case of primary obsessional slowness, the patient took up to 6 hours to wash and dress himself before starting the day. He felt that he had to shave each separate hair on his face and that his shoe-laces had to be exactly equal in length and to be tied with a double knot in exactly the same way each day. His everyday cleaning and dressing was divided into numerous tiny compartments, and each one had to be completed correctly and in the same stereotyped fashion each day.

In primary obsessional slowness, the person rarely resists carrying out the actions in his compulsive, meticulous way. The disorder tends to develop in early adulthood and take a chronic course, leading to increasing degrees of incapacitation. The patients tend to be socially isolated.

Some general comments

Presence of more than one problem

It was noted earlier that most obsessive–compulsive patients have more than one type of problem (see Chapter 3). Washing and checking often coexist, as do other compulsions and obsessions. Furthermore, a patient with one major problem at the time of referral may well have had a different major problem, or problems, in the past. Even within the same problem, the details can change with time.

The significance of numbers

We noted that many patients engage in compulsive behaviour a specific number of times. This is particularly the case with checkers and those with various other repeating compulsions, but some washers and cleaners also have special numbers. In a good proportion of cases, the special number has some 'magical' significance–either negative or positive. The use of numbers also helps patients to remember how far they have reached. Although some patients can explain why a particular number has become significant—e.g. the number of brothers and sisters, birth order, husband's/wife's birthday—others cannot.

Avoidance as the main problem

In some cases, the main feature may be not any active compulsive action, but avoidance of something, such as a certain number or a certain colour. In an earlier section we referred to a young woman who avoided the number four in every possible way (see pp. 54–55)—she did not have any active compulsive rituals, either overt or mental. Some patients with severe obsessive–compulsive disorders avoid washing, checking, or changing their clothes, since the activity in question involves exhausting rituals and takes up a great deal of time. Patients with severe contamination fears try to avoid coming into contact with others, leading a reclusive-like life, feeling safe only in their homes, in some cases only in their bedrooms. Howard Hughes, mentioned earlier (pp. 46–47), had an existence marked by such extensive avoidance in the later years of his life.

Indecisiveness

A feature seen in many obsessive–compulsive patients is indecisiveness. This is particularly so for checkers, whose obsessions often appear in the form of doubts, for hoarders, and for many of those with other kinds of compulsions. Having to make a decision often triggers off doubting and related checking and other compulsive behaviour in these patients. In severe cases, the difficulty in making decisions renders the patient inactive—the difficulty is not confined to major decisions, but occurs in trivial day-to-day matters. For example, one female patient found getting dressed in the morning almost impossible because she could not decide what clothes to wear. She would put on, and then take off, several dresses. Eventually, her mother had to decide each night what the woman should wear the next day; all her other clothes were locked away at night. Another patient had virtually given up shopping for groceries because she had such agonizing difficulty in deciding which articles to purchase. It could take her up to 15 minutes to decide which cereal to select, and extra time to select the particular box of cereal.

Perfectionism

In a proportion of obsessive–compulsive patients, striving for perfection is a feature of their difficulties. They feel tense and unhappy unless something is done 'perfectly'; and, as a result, they often find they repeat things incessantly (e.g. writing a letter), and often do not manage to finish a job at all. One female patient, who was doing advanced work at a university, came for help because she was not making any progress with her research. Every sentence was 'imperfect', and she could not proceed with the work until she got a 'perfect' sentence, a 'perfect' paragraph, and so on. She had been 'writing' this report for years, yet there was little she could show as a tangible product. Her supervisors were sympathetic, but baffled by her difficulty.

Scrupulosity

Some people with obsessive–compulsive disorder are exceedingly scrupulous. They feel a compulsion to tell the complete truth, and do so repeatedly and in great detail, even when listeners show no interest or express impatience. The word 'scrupulosity' is derived from the Latin *scrupus,* a pebble, and a similarity is implied between the insistent need to remove an irritating pebble from one's shoe and the insistent need to be completely truthful and completely honest. A troubling thought or urge is like having a pebble in one's shoe, a 'mental irritant'. The repeated 'confessions' almost invariably involve moral issues and moral doubts. A salesman of electrical goods felt compelled to inform customers of all of the potential dangers and limitations of the equipment he was supposed to be selling; in some instances he even visited customers at their homes to reiterate the limitations of equipment that they had bought from him. Affected people feel uneasy and unsettled by their moral/religious doubts and possible misdemeanours, however trivial, and feel compelled to disclose them, to 'confess'. They generally obtain transitory relief but in compulsive scrupulosity the removal of one mental irritant, one pebble, soon leads to its replacement by a new irritant.

One patient felt compelled repeatedly to tell her relations about her few and trivial amorous indiscretions, despite their disinterest, and when their patience came to an end, she tried telling her friends and, ultimately, her colleagues. Another patient felt compelled to report to the police station whenever she heard of a serious local crime because she was troubled by the possibility that she was responsible for the crime, even though she could not remember the precise details of her actions. When the local police recognized her psychological problem and expressed impatience with her visits, she travelled to a fresh police station to make her confession. This progression continued until she was travelling to police stations that were over 100 miles from her home. Like other people with compulsive scrupulosity, she had an over-developed conscience. Some famous religious figures, such as John Bunyan, Martin Luther, and St. Therese, gave vivid descriptions of the torments of their extreme scrupolosity, and, in these instances and others, the 'pebbles' were repugnant, recurring sinful thoughts.

Scrupulosity is related to an inflated sense of responsibility, and in these case illustrations the patients were burdened by inappropriately wide and inflated feelings of responsibility.

4

Effects on family, work, and social life

🔁 Key points

- The considerable effects of obsessive–compulsive disorders on family life are described.

- These effects are magnified when the patient has a severe form of the disorder.

- Most families strive to find a middle way between emotional support for the affected person and setting firm limits on the extent to which the household is dominated by the wishes and needs of the patient.

- There are no golden rules for families to follow in helping an affected member of the family, and each family has to tailor their arrangements according to the structure and routines of the household, while trying to ensure that the patient receives expert professional help.

- In severe cases the patient may be incapable of working, but most people with mild obsessive–compulsive disorder continue with their normal working life.

- Similarly, the social life of a severely affected patient is likely to be minimal, but mild cases can participate fully in social life.

- Obsessive–compulsive disorders often place a strain on marriages, and can lead to separations.

- ◆ The marriage and reproduction rates of severe cases of obsessive–compulsive disorder are well below the average.

- ◆ Some forms of obsessive–compulsive disorder interfere with a satisfactory sexual life, but most patients continue to engage in sexual activity.

How the family is affected

Obsessive–compulsive disorders usually have a significant effect on the other members of a patient's family. It is a puzzling disorder and the affected families struggle to find the best way to help their son, daughter, or spouse. Why does this rational person repeatedly engage in persistent and unadaptive checking, washing, cleaning, and avoidance—even though he recognizes that his behaviour is irrational and extreme? Why can't he control *this* behaviour as he controls most of his other behaviour? What exactly does he mean when he says he is 'compelled' to wash, clean, and check over and over again? How can we help him? What should we do?

There is no golden rule for family members to follow; the problems faced by each family are distinctive. In principle, however, it is advisable to provide emotional support and encouragement to obtain treatment, but to refrain from being drawn into the patient's rituals and compulsions. In many instances this can be difficult, and minor compromises are almost unavoidable. However, a search for the precisely 'correct' way of dealing with all of the problems that arise can end in frustration. It is best to bear in mind that there is no golden rule.

Families are affected in a number of ways. In some cases, the patient may consistently turn to a family member for reassurance, asking questions such as: 'Did I do it right?', 'Do you think I am going mad?', 'Are you sure I did it?', 'Is it really safe?', and so on. In most cases, the relatives provide reassurance despite the tiresome nature of the repeated questions. In some cases, family members are requested to carry out some compulsive activities (such as extreme cleaning) on the patient's behalf. In others, the patient may demand that others in the family follow certain rules of behaviour, and get angry if they do not comply; for example, changing from their outdoor clothing to indoor clothing immediately they return home. The use of the bathroom is a common source of disagreement and annoyance.

Some patients dominate their families in a remarkable manner. A cleaner with an obsession about dirt may prohibit family members from entering the house with their shoes on, insist on everyone washing their hands and clothes at a certain frequency, totally bar them from certain parts of the house, and impose all sorts of other restrictions. In one case, the patient allowed only a very narrow path through the main lounge, next to the wall, for family members to walk on and—to make matters worse—they had to do this without touching or brushing against the wall. They also had to keep their towels in polythene bags to avoid them coming into contact with the patient's own towels. One mother did not let her children or husband use the bathroom or kitchen in the morning until she had properly cleaned and washed these places, which took a good deal of time. As a result of this, on many days the husband was late going to work and the children were late for school. Another woman did not cook for her family on most days, since she had failed to clean the kitchen and the utensils satisfactorily in time; so they had to eat out or order take-away meals. A divorced woman got married for the second time, but would not let her new husband into her house in case he brought in contamination from outside. In extreme cases the patient feels that the home is so irredeemably contaminated that the family must move; the first move is not infrequently followed by the need for a second move even farther away, and even to a new city.

Some children of obsessive–compulsive patients are made to abide by all sorts of restrictions. They may have cleaning and washing rituals imposed on them, or have to do everything according to a fixed routine and/or avoid an extensive list of potential contaminants. Visits from friends may be disallowed. When they return from school or play, they may be made to remove their outer clothes and put them into laundry bags before entering the house. One woman insisted on bathing each of her children every morning, and this was done in a rigid, ritualistic manner: each child was bathed in turn, washing certain parts of the body first, other parts next, and so on, and then dried with a certain number of towels. Another mother did not allow her son to go anywhere near her husband when he returned from work, until he had a shower and donned fresh 'indoor' clothes. This eventually led to a major marital conflict and the couple separated.

Why do spouses, cohabitees, parents, children, and other relatives tolerate their lives being disrupted and controlled to such a degree by a patient? Many respond to the patient's requests and demands initially with questioning or refusal, but in the end give up and begin to comply for the sake of peace. Some family members say that they comply with the wishes of the patient out of love and kindness ('She cannot help it').

However, many relatives refuse to comply with the patient's requests, despite quarrels and tantrums. In some families, one key member may comply while another is totally unyielding. A teenage girl always received reassurance from her mother about all sorts of doubts and worries she had, but the father never gave her any kind of reassurance. Her mother also complied with numerous demands, keeping the kitchen door open in a certain way, the clock kept facing a particular direction, windows kept open at a certain angle, and so on. The father, however, always refused to comply. This led to the girl's problems causing major conflict within the family.

A mother's account

The following account, given by the mother of a 17-year-old girl with severe obsessive–compulsive problems, illustrates the way in which a patient with this disorder can drastically affect the family.

 Family member's perspective

Jenny would get very upset if her things were touched by any of us—even accidentally... . Her towel is kept well away from the other towels in the bathroom, her soap is kept separate, and her toilet paper is kept in a paper bag, separate. She insists on the bathroom being thoroughly cleaned by one of us before she goes in, and she spends hours in the bathroom, washing and washing.

Jenny's chair at the dining table is kept covered with a sheet and her plate, mug, and cutlery are kept separate in a drawer. She will eat with us, but not if Ken (her brother) is there. She gets worse when Ken is at home. She says it is not really him but his girlfriend Carol that upsets her. She thinks that this girl somehow makes things dirty, including Ken, and that the whole house is affected. She wouldn't let Ken touch her things at all. Carol is not allowed to come into the house now. Anything sent by her is taboo. She didn't even open the Christmas present that Ken gave her, as she felt that it would somehow make her dirty, as Ken had been to see Carol that day. Now Ken stays away much of the time, and doesn't bring Carol here any more. Poor girl, she is not dirty at all. We all like her, but Jenny won't let us invite her or welcome her. Carol understands and so does Ken, but he still gets very angry sometimes. Some days ago he threatened to bring Carol home for the day. Jenny made such a scene; she said she would leave home for good. In the end, we all felt that Carol should not come... . But it is not only Carol and things to do with her. That is the worst, but Jenny thinks most things are dirty. She hardly leaves her room now. Most things in the house she won't go near... .

She gets me to wash her clothes separately from the others and to dry them separately. You can't reason with her. She gets very upset, or very angry. Once, she made me wash the seats of the car because I had given lift to someone. We are all sorry for her, but we just don't know what to do

Effects on work and social life

The occupational and social effects of an obsessive–compulsive disorder depend on the severity of the problem. In mild to moderate cases, patients are usually able to continue working and maintain a reasonable social life. However, in severe cases, the social and occupational effects of the disorder can be incapacitating.

Many patients manage to continue working by successfully concealing their problems. It is slowness and checking, and related doubting, that is most likely to affect an obsessive–compulsive person's occupational effectiveness. Their efficiency may gradually become noticeably impaired. A patient with primary obsessional slowness, who required many hours to get ready in the morning, found it increasingly hard to arrive for work on time. He tried to deal with this by waking up earlier and earlier, but eventually he could not keep his job.

Among people who labour under an inflated sense of responsibility, there is a strong tendency to resist any increases in responsibility at work, even to the extent of repeatedly refusing promotion.

Those with washing and cleaning problems may try to find an office or desk close to the washroom. Their frequent visits to the washroom, or their habit of wiping their desk clean with a wet wipe each morning, may be noticed by colleagues. One woman kept changing jobs every few months. She eventually divulged to a therapist the reason for her job changes. The moment she was convinced that office colleagues had noticed her frequent hand-washing and cleaning rituals, she would look for new employment. As she was quite an efficient employee, she had no difficulty in getting jobs.

Students with severe obsessive–compulsive problems encounter considerable difficulties in their studies. Ruminations may take up a lot of time, as in the case described on p. 26. Repeated checking can sometimes make progress with assignments, or even reading, quite a struggle. As noted above (p. 61) an advanced student made no progress with the writing of her major report because of severe perfectionism. One male student who feared contamination from others gradually stopped going to class, or even to the university library.

If a person spends a great deal of time checking or cleaning, or engaging in compulsive rituals, he has correspondingly less time, or indeed inclination, to engage in social activities. If the disorder is severe, their social life is restricted. Avoidance of certain places and certain behaviour (e.g. hand-shaking) out of fear of contamination can understandably lead to a reduction in social contact. Severe fear of contamination can also lead to visitors being disallowed because they might bring germs or dirt into the house.

Sex and marriage

The disorder can place an enormous strain on married life. The divorce and separation rates are high for people affected by this disorder, among the highest of any group with psychological or psychiatric problems. If the problem centres on contamination from bodily products, it is common to find associated sexual problems. For example, a wife may demand a state of extreme cleanliness before sexual relations, and insist on elaborate washing and cleaning rituals after intercourse. In some, sex may be restricted to one room or one part of a room that is kept almost clinically clean in order to prevent contamination from seminal fluid. In some cases, such concerns can lead to a total inability to engage in sexual activity. One patient felt that he should have sexual contact only on certain days of the month, linked to the significance he attached to particular numbers. He would often invent excuses to avoid intimate contact on other days. It was after more than 2 years of marriage, and much unhappiness, that he told his wife the truth.

In severe cases of obsessive–compulsive disorder, marital and sexual problems are common. However, in the majority of cases the disorder does not impede the patient's sex life.

5

Prevalence and related factors

➡ Key points

◆ Obsessive–compulsive disorders are not common.

◆ A high proportion of clinical cases are severe.

◆ Many people who experience obsessions and/or engage in compulsions are not distressed or disabled by them, and neither need nor seek professional help.

◆ Some cases emerge in childhood, but the large majority develop in late adolescence or early adulthood.

◆ Obsessive–compulsive disorders seldom develop late in life.

◆ Depression and/or stress can provoke or exacerbate obsessive–compulsive disorders.

◆ Obsessive–compulsive disorders occur in many parts of the world, but the particular features of the disorder tend to be influenced by cultural beliefs and practices.

How common is obsessive–compulsive disorder?

Obsessive–compulsive disorders are comparatively rare, but not as rare as was believed many years ago. Early estimates of the occurrence of the disorder in the general population, thought to be about 0.05%—i.e. 1 out of every 2000—were too low. In part this under-estimation reflected ignorance about obsessive–compulsive disorders, and more recent surveys indicate that the likelihood of developing the disorder sometime during a person's life is closer to 1.6%. This estimate comes from a large US national survey carried out in 2001–03, involving over 9000 people in various communities. By comparison, the likelihood of developing a depressive disorder is 16.6%, and the likelihood of a social phobia is 12.1%. However, a disproportionately large percentage of the cases of obsessive–compulsive disorder fall into the severe category (roughly 50%). In sum, obsessive–compulsive disorders are not very common but a majority of them are severe. Only one-quarter fall into the mild category.

Among psychiatric out-patients, fewer than 1% suffer from this disorder. Among in-patients the figure is higher, but certainly under 5%. There are, however, problems with figures such as these, since diagnostic practices are not consistent across clinics and hospitals.

It should be mentioned that many people have obsessions and/or compulsions that do not cause sufficient distress or interference with their lives to warrant diagnosing them as clinical cases of obsessive–compulsive disorder. Even among those whose problems do amount to clinical disorder, a proportion of them never seek help; in fact, some positively conceal their problems.

Sex and age

There is no clear preponderance of either males or females among adult patients with obsessive–compulsive disorder. In child obsessive–compulsive disorder, the prevalence is higher for boys (see Chapter 9). There are, however, sex differences in some of the clinical groups within the disorder, which have already been mentioned.

The onset of obsessive–compulsive disorder is usually in adolescence or early adulthood. Most cases emerge before the age of 25. In one large series of patients seen in a London hospital, in 92% of the cases the disorder had started between the ages of 10 and 40. The onset tends to be earlier in males than in females. It is rare for someone to develop the disorder for the first time after the age of 45. By the age of 30, nearly three-quarters of all identified cases have been diagnosed. A considerable time may elapse before the affected person comes to a clinic or hospital, although prolonged delays are becoming less common. The problem is more readily recognized than it was two or three decades ago, and the recent expansion of psychological services in the UK promises to improve the recognition and early treatment of obsessive–compulsive and other anxiety disorders.

Marriage, family, social class, and education

Many studies show that a high proportion of adult obsessive–compulsive patients are not married and that there is a greater tendency for male patients to be single than female patients. These patients tend to get married at a later age than most, including other psychiatric patients. There is also evidence that these patients have fewer children.

It used to be believed by clinicians that obsessive–compulsive disorders are more common among those in higher social classes and with a higher educational background. However, the results of the large community study carried out in the USA between 2001 and 2003 failed to support this belief.

Course of the disorder

In roughly half of all cases, the problems begin and develop gradually. Among those with an acute onset, there is a preponderance of washers and cleaners, over checkers. Generally, the course of the disorder shows some fluctuation. There may be periods when the problem is clearly present and active, followed by relatively good periods. These relatively good periods are, however, not fully symptom-free in most cases. In some cases, perhaps about half, there is steady worsening of the disorder. We have already noted (see pp. 27–28) that the problems get worse with depression. Also, when the person is under stress, the chances of obsessions and compulsions reappearing, or getting worse, are increased.

Factors that contribute to obsessive–compulsive disorder

It is difficult to give a definitive account of the factors that contribute to the origins of the disorder, since the information available is too limited. Data from patients are mostly retrospective, and not sufficiently accurate.

Precipitating events and stress

Even in cases where a specific time of onset can be traced, a single clear precipitating event is not always found. However, among those where there is a single event preceding the disorder, the onset can be sudden and dramatic—onset within a matter of days or even hours of the precipitating event is not unknown. In one case, a man developed severe obsessive–compulsive problems related to fear of illness immediately after undergoing surgery for the removal of a non-malignant growth. In another, a woman who was brutally sexually assaulted while on holiday abroad found herself thoroughly and repeatedly cleaning herself and throwing away the things she had with her at the time. This rapidly developed into full-blown contamination fears and extensive washing and cleaning rituals. In an earlier chapter (see pp. 31–32) we noted that a small proportion of patients who develop post-traumatic stress disorder after a catastrophic experience may also develop clinically significant obsessive–compulsive problems.

Cases of clear and dramatic onset linked to a severely traumatic personal experience are not very common. On the other hand, stressful experiences of various sorts in the period of time preceding a more gradual onset of the disorder are frequently reported. These include emotional problems in relationships, overwork, pregnancy and childbirth, problems in marriage or sex life, illness, and death or illness of a close relative. In a significant minority of cases, the onset of obsessive–compulsive disorder is preceded by an episode of depression.

There are no known links between the nature of onset and outcome, and no known link between the type of precipitating event and outcome.

Parental influence

Are there parental influences? If a child grows up in a household where one of the parents is severely affected by obsessive–compulsive disorder, is it likely that he will also develop the same problem? Many children briefly display comparable behaviour, but very few develop obsessive–compulsive disorders. Children of an affected parent seldom develop lasting, specific compulsive behaviour. If anything, they are more likely to develop over-dependence and timidity.

Heredity

What about genetic factors—is the disorder inherited? The kinds of studies that are needed to answer this question conclusively do not exist. Of the available twin studies, comparing the occurrence of the disorder in pairs of identical (monozygotic) twins with the occurrence in non-identical (dizygotic) twins, some appear to suggest a higher rate of concordance (i.e. both twins in a pair having the disorder) for identical pairs, while others have reported different findings. The same applies to studies of family members. A study carried out in London, which compared the first-degree relatives (father, mother, brother, sister, son, daughter) of 50 obsessive–compulsive patients with those of a matched group who did not have the disorder, showed that the former group had a higher rate of lifetime psychiatric problems—i.e. the relatives of the obsessive–compulsive patients had more psychiatric disorders in general at some time in their life, than did the relatives of the comparison group. However, no greater incidence of obsessive–compulsive disorder itself was found among this group.

Taken together, the available studies suggest that there is a genetic contribution, but that this does not make someone specifically vulnerable to obsessive–compulsive disorders. What appears to be inherited is a general emotional oversensitivity, which can predispose one to the development of some form of anxiety disorder.

Culture and obsessive–compulsive disorder

Obsessive–compulsive disorders are found in different parts of the world, and in different cultural settings. Descriptions are available for most Western cultures, as well as India, Pakistan, Hong Kong, Japan, Taiwan, Egypt, Singapore, and Sri Lanka, among others. The similarities of the obsessions and compulsions found in diverse countries are remarkable; the features reported in a large series of obsessive–compulsive patients in India were not very different from those found in studies in the UK or the USA.

A very early Buddhist text has an interesting account of a monk at the time of Buddha (over 25 centuries ago), who engaged in what can only be described as compulsive behaviour. It was reported that a monk, called Sammunjani, spent most of his time sweeping the monastery with a broom and that this activity took priority over everything else. The Japanese Zen master Hakuin (1685–1768), a major figure in the history of Zen Buddhism, was described as having suffered from severe obsessive–compulsive problems as a young man. The main feature of this appears to have been obsessional thoughts in the form of doubts.

This period in the life of Hakuin, who was a major religious leader in the Far East, bears interesting comparison with one stage of the life of an even more influential religious leader in the West, Martin Luther. Luther (1483–1543) was tormented by recurrent and severe doubts and intrusive, blasphemous thoughts. He was assailed by doubts about whether or not he had carried out all sorts of acts that were sinful, and persistently doubted whether he had confessed fully and properly. During extreme periods he confessed several times each day.

Similar unwanted intrusive thoughts of a blasphemous nature also affected John Bunyan (1628–1688), the author of *Pilgrim's progress*. He gave a vivid account of these in his autobiographical book *Grace abounding to the chief of sinners*, which was first published in 1666. One of his great fears was that, instead of words of praise, he might betray God and utter terrible and blasphemous accusations against Him. He was extremely distressed by these unwanted thoughts and tried very hard to resist them. In a particularly informative passage, Bunyan describes his struggles with one of his unwanted thoughts in these words:

> But it was neither my dislike of the thought, nor yet any desire and endeavour to resist it, that at the least did shake or abate the continuation of force and strength thereof; for it did always in almost whatever I thought, intermix itself with, in such sort that I could neither eat my food, stoop for a pin, chop a stick, or cast mine eye to look on this or that, but still the temptation would come, *Sell Christ for this, or Sell Christ for that; sell him, sell him.*

The phenomena of obsessions and compulsions are not confined to one culture or one period of time. The basic features are essentially the same across diverse cultural backgrounds and eras. The specific contents of the obsessions, however, can reflect common concerns found in a particular culture or era. For example, obsessions and compulsions related to fears of contamination by asbestos was a relatively common problem among patients with obsessive–compulsive disorder in Britain 20–30 years ago. In recent years, there has been an increase in obsessions, and associated compulsions, pertaining to the threat of HIV/AIDS.

Another way in which culture has some influence on the nature of obsessive–compulsive disorder is religion. The content of a patient's obsessions can reflect religious beliefs and ideas. Studies in India have shown a preponderance of obsessive–compulsive disorder with themes of dirt and contamination among Hindu patients; this is seen as reflecting the preoccupation with matters of purity and cleanliness in that culture. A study from Israel, looking at obsessive–compulsive symptoms in a sample of 34 patients, found symptoms linked to religious practices in 13 out of 19 ultra-orthodox Jewish patients, but in only 1 out of 15 non-ultra-orthodox Jewish patients. Further, those with strong religious beliefs appear to be prone to developing clinical obsessions as a result of attaching excessive personal significance to unwanted intrusive thoughts. Blasphemous or sexual thoughts, for example, may cause a lot of distress in those brought up in a strict religious background. This distress can then lead to the perpetuation of the thought, turning it into a clinically significant obsession.

Obsessions and compulsions across the age spectrum

The elderly

While the onset of obsessive–compulsive disorder is uncommon in elderly people, there are exceptions. A small number of people may develop the disorder at a late age. Also some, with an earlier onset, continue to suffer from obsessive–compulsive disorder into old age. Recent reports show that some elderly patients have obsessional thoughts that reflect concerns related to their stage in life.

One patient, in his early seventies, had the recurrent thought: 'What will happen to me when Phyllis dies?'. Phyllis was, of course, his wife, and she was 8 years younger. The patient knew that the chances of her dying before him were not high, and he was fully aware that his thoughts were irrational. He also had a vivid, terrifying visual image of his wife dying, which often accompanied the thought. He reported that the thought came to him over a hundred times a day. He was very distressed by this and sought help.

Other cases of elderly patients with similar obsessions have also been reported. The relatively small literature on this subject shows two recurrent themes in obsessive–compulsive problems in old age. One relates to aspects of physical functioning, the other to religious and moral concerns.

Children and adolescents

Obsessive–compulsive disorder can occur in childhood and adolescence, and there is a growing literature on this subject. A discussion of childhood obsessive–compulsive disorder is provided in Chapter 9.

6

Theories and explanations

➜ Key points

◆ At present there is no comprehensive explanation of obsessive–compulsive disorder.

◆ The learning theory explanation proposed that the disorder results from maladaptive learning and adverse life experiences, but was too general.

◆ Nevertheless it produced a psychological treatment, behaviour therapy, that is moderately effective.

◆ A modern expansion of the theory, cognitive theory, places great emphasis on the person's beliefs, interpretations of events, thoughts, and images, and led to the development of improved treatment—cognitive behaviour therapy.

◆ According to cognitive theory, people who develop obsessive–compulsive disorder suffer from an extremely inflated sense of responsibility, and inflated estimations of the probability and severity of disastrous events.

◆ A considerable amount of research is being carried out on the cognitive theory and the derived treatment technique, cognitive behaviour therapy.

◆ One of the earliest psychological explanations of obsessive–compulsive disorder was derived from psychoanalysis, but research failed to support the theory, and psychoanalytic therapy is no longer recommended.

- ◆ Biological theories of obsessive–compulsive disorder are widely discussed, and a prominent view is that the disorder results from a biochemical imbalance in the brain.

- ◆ Biological theories are associated with the use of medications, especially anti-depressant drugs.

- ◆ The medications often are helpful, particularly when the patient is significantly depressed.

- ◆ There are no laboratory tests for obsessive–compulsive disorder.

Different theories have been put forward in attempts to explain obsessive–compulsive disorder. It is not possible, in a short book like this, to attempt a full discussion of these theories. What we shall do in this chapter, instead, is to take a brief look at some of them.

Psychological perspectives

The learning view

An influential psychological approach proposes that obsessive–compulsive disorders, and other neurotic problems, are the result of maladaptive learning; they are predominantly acquired by life experiences. This approach is also referred to as the behavioural view. A person may learn, through association with a painful, threatening, or upsetting experience, to become extremely anxious about certain situations, or objects, or people. He may also learn that certain behaviour reduces the anxiety, and, as a result, this behaviour becomes strengthened. For example, compulsive washing behaviour reduces the fear of contamination, and therefore becomes established and strengthened. Whenever the person feels contaminated he engages in the compulsive washing as a prompt and reasonably reliable way of reducing or preventing the fear.

There is evidence that, in most cases, carrying out of the compulsive behaviour does indeed reduce anxiety or discomfort. Experimental evidence from studies of animals and humans also provides some support for the learning theory view. In aversive situations, animals engage in previously learned anxiety-reducing behaviour in a stereotyped, repetitive way, even though this behaviour does not lead to escape or relief from the current situation. This suggests that in stressful situations, previously useful anxiety-reducing behaviour may be rigidly resorted to, even though it has no logical relationship to the present stress. The seemingly senseless ritualistic behaviour of some obsessive–compulsive patients is construed as a similar phenomenon—in an aversive situation they resort to previously developed stereotyped behaviour that brings temporary relief.

However, the learning view has difficulty in providing a comprehensive explanation of these problems. As we noted earlier (p. 71), many patients with obsessive–compulsive disorder do not recall any initial painful experience or experiences as the starting point of their problems; i.e. there is no clear direct learning experience. Also, the theory gives no adequate explanation as to why only particular kinds of items (dirt, germs, and so on) acquire frightening qualities and lead to obsessions and compulsions. It has been suggested that there are certain 'prepared fears', namely that we are primed to acquire fears that have biological significance. The learning theory is unable to explain disorders that are primarily cognitive. For example, it is silent about the origin and nature of obsessions, and about primary slowness, and is not helpful in explaining compulsive hoarding.

The cognitive behavioural view

A theoretical account that adds a cognitive component to the learning (behavioural) view has been developed in recent years. This approach takes into account the person's cognitions—beliefs, thoughts, images, etc.—as an important aspect of the problem. It is noted that many patients have an exaggerated appraisal of risk and danger. Many also have a greatly exaggerated sense of being personally responsible for avoiding/preventing harm and disaster. The way one appraises one's own thoughts and images is seen as contributing to the development of the disorder. There are indications that this new, expanded account will lead to better understanding and improved results. Already two detailed and specific cognitive theories have been developed, one to account for obsessions and the other for compulsive checking.

There is sound evidence that cognitive behaviour therapy is an effective psychological treatment for obsessive–compulsive disorder, and it is accordingly recommended by the National Centre for Health and Clinical Excellence (NICE). Some problems remain to be sorted out, and too large a number of patients decline the treatment or drop-out prematurely. Methods for treating mental contamination are at the development stage.

Reference is made to the cognitive behavioural approach in various parts of this book.

The psychoanalytical view

The earliest psychological theory is the psychoanalytical one. Psychoanalysis is a treatment technique for neurotic disorders that was developed by Sigmund Freud, and the rationale for the treatment is provided by his elaborate psychoanalytical theory. There are also derivatives of psychoanalytic treatment, broadly classed as psychodynamic therapy.

In the psychoanalytic approach, obsessions and compulsions are seen as symptoms of some deeper problem in the person's unconscious mind. Certain memories, desires, and conflicts are kept out of consciousness, or repressed, because they would otherwise cause anxiety. These repressed elements may later manifest themselves as neurotic symptoms. Fixation (or 'getting stuck') at a particular stage of development, caused by various factors during one's formative years, determines the nature of the neurotic symptoms that appear in later life. The compulsions are viewed as defensive reactions that suppress the real, hidden anxieties. The theory was not supported by satisfactory research.

There is no evidence that psychoanalytical treatment is effective for this disorder. The NICE report states that psychoanalysis is not recommended for the treatment of obsessive–compulsive disorders.

Biological causation

Within the past few decades, it has been suggested by several authors that obsessive–compulsive disorders are caused by a biological disturbance. The biological theory proposes that the disorder is caused by a biochemical imbalance in the brain—in particular, it has been claimed that obsessive–compulsive disorder arises because of an inadequate supply of serotonin. (Serotonin is a neurotransmitter—i.e. a chemical substance that carries messages between cells in the brain. It is known that serotonin plays an important part in brain functioning.) This theory originally emerged from the finding that an anti-depressive drug, clomipramine, which blocks the natural loss of serotonin, can produce therapeutic effects in these patients.

The biological theory has gained some support, but has also been criticized. Therapeutic improvements of equal or greater magnitude than those produced by clomipramine or similar drugs have been achieved through purely psychological treatment methods—when the serotonin level is ignored. There is no evidence that people suffering from obsessive–compulsive disorder have serotonin levels that differ from those of people suffering from other comparable psychological disorders, especially other anxiety disorders, or levels that differ from people free of any such disorder. Furthermore, there is no relationship between the amount of clomipramine absorbed and the degree of therapeutic change. Even with high doses of the drug, and hence high levels of serotonin, relatively few patients are free of obsessive–compulsive symptoms, and some patients do not respond. It has also been found that the patient's initial response to clomipramine does not provide a good basis for predicting the longer term effects of this medication. Additionally, on present evidence, one of the most effective anti-obsessive drugs is clomipramine, which is even more effective than comparable drugs that are more effective in boosting the levels of serotonin.

Theories of biological causation do not provide an explanation for the different forms of obsessive–compulsive disorder. They are too general and are non-specific. To illustrate this problem, questions about why one person develops compulsive washing and another develops compulsive hoarding or obsessions are not addressed.

Another problem with the biological theory is that the attempt to derive the cause of a disorder from a therapeutic effect is risky. For example, the fact that aspirin relieves a headache tells us little about the cause of the headache, and it certainly does not tell us that the headache occurred because the person was short of aspirin. The fact that clomipramine often reduces obsessive–compulsive symptoms does not mean that the disorder was caused by a shortage of clomipramine, or of the serotonin that it bolsters.

It is common for patients to receive medications before and during psychological treatment, and treatments such as cognitive behaviour therapy are effective for a majority of patients with or without medications. In severe cases, especially those who are significantly depressed, medications are commonly used in advance of psychological treatment.

A great deal of research is being carried out at present on this issue. No doubt, in the next few years important new information about the biological theory will be available. The evidence supporting the theory is not conclusive at present.

Other approaches

Some writers have offered the view that obsessive–compulsive patients' problems are the result of a cognitive defect—i.e. a deficit in their thinking, or thinking style. It is usually assumed that these putative deficits are biological.

Many patients, especially those struggling with compulsive checking, complain of a failing memory and/or an inability to attend satisfactorily. When engaged in repeated checking, it is common for patients to experience difficulty in remembering how many times they have checked and whether or not they checked satisfactorily. These complaints can be interpreted as indicating the presence of a memory/attention defect. However, the available evidence is too weak to support the view that a cognitive defect or an impaired cognitive style is the explanation of this disorder. Moreover, it has been shown in several experiments that patients with obsessive–compulsive disorder have a *superior* memory for events and items that are particularly significant for them (e.g. remembering precisely which items were contaminated years ago), and that their general ability to remember is normal when assessed by standard measures of memory. It is likely that their complaints are evidence of a distrust of their memory and attention rather than a cognitive defect.

Conclusions

Our understanding of obsessive–compulsive disorders is steadily improving but at present there is no comprehensive explanation for obsessive–compulsive disorders. It is possible that different aspects of the problem require different explanations. Of the currently available theories, the cognitive behavioural one is the most promising, and explanations for specific forms of the disorder have been put forward (e.g. for obsessions and for compulsive checking). Further developments are awaited. It appears that many factors are involved in the genesis and persistence of this disorder. As noted previously (see pp. 72–73), genetic and family factors may make it more likely that someone develops these problems. It is also clear that stressful experiences probably play a very important part. There is substantial evidence that stressful emotional experiences can lead to recurrent intrusive unwanted thoughts and images. It has been suggested that when a traumatic or stressful experience is not fully emotionally processed—i.e. resolved or absorbed—it may leave residual effects that manifest themselves as various symptoms. In this way, recurrent intrusions that are normally short-lived may become chronic and persistent in some people. Some recent clinical reports document the development of the disorder following a seriously traumatic experience in some people (see pp. 31–32), and we know that victims of sexual assault are at some risk for the development of symptoms of obsessive–compulsive disorder.

The absence of a comprehensive explanation of the disorder at present does not mean that effective treatments are not available. As with many other clinical problems, the development of treatments for obsessive–compulsive disorder has far outpaced the development of explanations for why and how it occurs in certain people.

7

Treatment

> **➔ Key points**

- Obsessive–compulsive disorders are treated by psychological methods or medications, and, not infrequently, by a combination of the two.

- Psychological treatment, notably cognitive behaviour therapy, is effective in a majority of cases.

- The treatment generally requires up to 12 sessions, which last about 1 hour each.

- The treatment of severe cases usually requires more extensive therapy.

- A majority of severe cases are treated by medication prior to and/or during psychological treatment.

- Patients who are suffering from significant depression are likely to receive medication prior to and/or during psychological treatment.

- Psychological treatment in a group is effective for dealing with compulsions but the treatment of obsessions is more effective when provided individually.

- Medications often are effective but may need to be continued over a long period, and are prone to produce some side-effects.

Many patients with obsessive–compulsive disorders can now be treated successfully, in contrast to the situation even as recently as the 1960s, when little could be done to help them. This change has been brought about mainly by the development of the psychological treatment, behaviour therapy, later expanded into cognitive behaviour therapy. This treatment method has been shown to be effective in the management of obsessive–compulsive disorders, particularly those that are of mild to moderate severity. In severe cases, cognitive behaviour therapy often is used in combination with medication. The methods of treatment are constantly being refined and improved. With increased understanding, the methods are becoming more specific and match the treatment to the particular manifestations of the disorder.

What is cognitive behaviour therapy?

Cognitive behaviour therapy combines two types of treatment: behaviour therapy and cognitive therapy. The method known as behaviour therapy was developed on the basis of hundreds of studies of how changes take place in human and animal behaviour. This knowledge was then used to establish methods for changing unadaptive and distressing human behaviour, such as intense fears, and was later expanded into cognitive behaviour therapy. In the 1950s, a South African doctor, Joseph Wolpe (1915–97), who later practised in Temple University, Philadelphia, introduced a technique for overcoming anxiety and fears. It consisted of systematically reducing the fears by a gradual and progressive method of 'desensitization', i.e. by reducing the person's sensitivity to whatever cues or situations provoked the fear. The patients were trained in self-relaxation, and during periods of induced deep relaxation they were repeatedly exposed to the frightening cue (e.g. a snake), for gradually increasing periods, and at gradually closer distances. In this way the patients became less and less sensitive to the frightening cue. Dr Wolpe then discovered that patients could be desensitized if they repeatedly formed images of the frightening cues or situations while in a state of deep relaxation. For example, they would repeatedly imagine a snake for say 2 minutes, while in a state of relaxation, and, after many such exercises they were less sensitive to the images of the snake, and, later, to actual snakes. This process of desensitization was refined over the years and planned, repeated, graded exposures to fearful cues, such as 'contaminated' items, was shaped into a successful technique for helping patients with obsessive–compulsive disorder.

The work of Professor Hans Eysenck (1916–97) in London contributed to the development and acceptance of behaviour therapy as a major approach to certain psychological problems. In essence, he said that many unadaptive behavioural problems are acquired by processes of learning—and what has been acquired by a learning process can be unlearned. Unadaptive behaviour falls into two categories: cases of faulty unadaptive learning, such as irrational fears, or problems that arise because of a failure to learn adaptive behaviour. In either case, it should be possible to correct matters by applying the principles of learning. The faulty learning can be undone, and new learning can be promoted. Therefore, behaviour therapy concentrated on the problem of behaviour itself. It did not assume, as the then prevalent psychoanalytical approach did, that patients' difficulties are symptoms of deeper unconscious complexes. Rather than attempting to unravel the putative deep causes, behaviour therapists worked directly on the problem behaviour. They concentrated more on the problem as it is now, and what factors are currently associated with it, rather than its past history. Of course, therapists need to know from the patient when the problem started, how it developed, and so on, but the main focus is on the problem as it is now, and therapist's efforts are geared towards modifying this problem.

The efficacy of behaviour therapy for a range of psychological disorders is well established, and the latest form—cognitive behaviour therapy—is now the psychological treatment of choice for obsessive–compulsive disorder, and other anxiety disorders. The independent NICE in the UK and the National Institute of Mental Health (NIMH) in the USA recommend cognitive behaviour therapy for obsessive–compulsive disorder. In their reports on obsessive–compulsive disorder, both of the institutes recommend this as a first-line treatment, and distinguish between the management of mild, moderate, and severe cases. In severe cases they recommend medications, and also cognitive behaviour therapy, as needed.

In recent years, behaviour therapy was expanded to include aspects of what is known as 'cognitive therapy'. The exclusive attention to problems of observable behaviour was found to be unnecessarily limited, and the therapy was expanded to include cognitions—thoughts, images ideas, beliefs, and attitudes. Cognitive therapists focus their treatment on eliciting the patient's cognitions that are relevant to his problems and on helping him to modify them. The most impressive work by cognitive therapists so far has been in the treatment of depression and panic. Depressed patients often have very negative thoughts, such as 'I am a worthless person', 'There is no point to my life', and so on. Attempts are made to modify these thoughts using a variety of techniques, including the elicitation of the reasons for continuing to endorse maladaptive beliefs, examining the evidence for the thoughts, assembling evidence that is inconsistent with them, and setting up behavioural tasks to gather disconfirming evidence. Cognitive therapy was originally developed for the treatment of depression but the concepts and techniques are now being used for other disorders as well, notably obsessive–compulsive disorder and panic disorder (see Rachman, S. and de Silva, P. (2004) *Panic disorder: the facts*, 2nd edn. Oxford University Press, Oxford).

The first part of this combined therapy is devoted to eliciting the patient's cognitions, especially those regarding their obsessive–compulsive disorder—beliefs, expectations, images, the nature of the person's estimations of risks and ultimate fears, their sense of personal responsibility, what has helped and why, what has failed and why, and so on. The patient's beliefs about risk, danger, and responsibility often play an important part in the disorder, and eliciting and helping to modify these is a key aspect of treatment.

An example of the value of the cognitive therapy can be illustrated by this case of a compulsive checker. In common with virtually all patients who struggle with their intense urges to check and repeatedly re-check, he had a grossly excessive sense of responsibility:

The patient believed that he was responsible for the safety and well-being of a wide range of people, and hence engaged in the excessive, repetitive checking of gas taps, electrical switches, and so on. Also, in common with other patients, he had a greatly inflated fear of making any errors, however trivial. Typically, he greatly over-estimated the probability of accidents or other misfortunes, and over-estimated the seriousness of any error or misfortune. The identification of this exaggerated sense of responsibility and a consideration of its irrationality and untoward consequences can be a most useful step in treatment. In his case, as the eldest of three children, he had been given family responsibilities from an early age because his father was alcohol dependent, aggressive, demanding, and incessantly critical. Even though the patient had his own family and very little contact with his father, he continued to feel under critical surveillance, and was highly vigilant every day, always keeping down any risks of errors. On occasions when he felt that he might have made an error, or overlooked a potential threat, he experienced fear. The cognitive analysis of his current fears suggested the probable origin of his obsessive–compulsive disorder and the reasons for its persistence. Much time and effort were put into distinguishing between the circumstances during his childhood and the punishments for 'errors', and those of his current life. The inflated feelings of responsibility, and his realistic responsibilities, were contrasted, but he nevertheless had difficulty in re-adjusting his feelings of responsibility. Progress was made, but an exclusive concentration on blocking his particular checking behaviour, without the cognitive analysis, would have been unsatisfactory.

Promising results have been obtained in the cognitive treatment of obsessions. This is unsurprising because obsessions are themselves cognitions, and earlier attempts to treat obsessions by introducing modifications of behaviour were not successful. It is said that the obsessions persist because the person attaches excessive personal significance to the unwanted, intrusive thoughts (e.g. 'having these thoughts means I am a sinful/dangerous person'). The therapeutic reduction of false appraisals can lead to great relief and improvement. This kind of cognitive work plays an important part in therapy for obsessive–compulsive patients.

Cognitive behaviour therapy continues to evolve, and significant advances are anticipated.

Exposure and response-prevention for those with observable compulsions

The application of behaviour therapy to obsessive–compulsive disorder goes back to the mid-1960s when a psychologist in London, Dr Victor Meyer, began to treat patients who had compulsive rituals with what became known as exposure and response-prevention (ERP). It consisted of two elements; arranging for the patient to enter the situations that made him feel anxious or very uncomfortable and triggered off his compulsive urges (exposure); and preventing the patient from carrying out his compulsive behaviour (response-prevention). This combination of real-life exposure plus response-prevention was established as a technique for treating patients with overt compulsive behaviour. Research in the UK, the USA, and The Netherlands led to improvements in the treatment and provided convincing evidence of its efficacy. It remains an important element in the treatment of patients who suffer from intense fears of contamination and observable compulsions.

Rationale

Before describing the details of this form of treatment, we need to mention the rationale behind it. Typically, an obsessive–compulsive patient with observable compulsions experiences fear/discomfort and a strong urge to carry out the compulsion when provoked by exposure to the trigger stimulus or situation (e.g. insecticides). When the patient engages in the compulsive behaviour, say hand-washing, the level of fear/discomfort generally declines somewhat. Naturally the patient recognizes the connection, and the resort to hand-washing is strengthened. As the decline in fear is at least moderate and fairly prompt, most patients come to believe that their fear/discomfort will continue until they carry out the relieving hand-wash. However, experiments have shown that the level of fear/discomfort, and the associated compulsive urges, usually decline spontaneously, even if the compulsive behaviour (e.g. washing) is not carried out. This natural decline occurs more slowly, between roughly 2 and 120 minutes, depending on the patient and stage of treatment. Early in treatment, the spontaneous decline can take up to 2 hours, but, as treatment progresses, the decline takes a few minutes. The spontaneous decline is demonstrated to the patient, and it is explained that if after an exposure to a fear cue, no compulsive behaviour is used to gain prompt relief, the fear and discomfort will fade out. Moreover, if this sequence of exposure and prevention of the compulsion is repeated many times, then the compulsion will weaken. After repeated sessions of ERP there is a cumulative effect, leading to the patient feeling progressively lower levels of discomfort and weaker urges to engage in the compulsive behaviour. The urges and fear/discomfort decline more easily and rapidly as treatment progresses.

The role of modelling

Modelling, a form of therapeutic imitation, is often used in the treatment programme, especially in the earliest stages. The therapist demonstrates to the patient how the exposures are done and how to inhibit the urges to carry out the relieving compulsion. For example, the therapist might touch the door handles, the floor, and so on, and then rub his hands together to spread the effect. After repeating the demonstration a few times the patient is encouraged to join in and copy the therapist's actions, or as many as he can manage.

The patient is asked to report the strength of the urges to carry out the compulsion (0–100) and the degree of fear/discomfort (0–100) that he feels after each exposure, and again after a few minutes have elapsed. Gradually the patient begins to experience the spontaneous decay of the urges and discomfort. Modelling can facilitate therapy, and often is needed to encourage a fearful patient to carry out certain required exercises. In many instances the patient will experience a slight reduction in fear from watching the therapist model carry out the simple exposure exercises, touching the door handles, floor, and so on. The modelling can be informative and motivating but is not an essential ingredient. The main component of the treatment is exposure and response-prevention.

Imaginal exposure

In some cases, imaginal exposure, also called 'exposure in fantasy', is used. When it is impractical to arrange exposures to the actual situation, such as public speaking, the patient is taught how to create vivid images as an alternative form of exposure. Some research suggests that for patients who fear that disasters may occur in the future, if they do not engage in their compulsions, imaginal exposure to these disasters may be a useful additional element in therapy. It is claimed that imaginal exposure can improve the long-term results of therapy, when used in addition to *in vivo* ERP, but its value remains to be confirmed.

Therapy in practice

How is the treatment done? It is important to stress that different therapists will set about their task in different ways, although the same principles are involved. This description should not be taken as a definitive account of precisely what all therapists do, but rather as an illustration of the general principles.

In the assessment, the therapist obtains detailed information from the patient about the full range of his difficulties. At this stage, the patient's beliefs and attitudes relevant to the problem are explored and discussed. The rationale for the treatment is provided, and often supplemented by written material. In treating mild cases, the course of therapy is short, say between four and eight sessions. Severe cases need more intensive and extensive therapy. In these cases, it is explained that the treatment can be difficult at times and that the patient retains overall control of the treatment programme. If ERP is to be used, he can slow it down, speed it up, or suggest changes in the order or content of exposure presentations. Patients are assured that no coercion is used at any time, and there will be no surprises. A description of ERP follows:

The therapist and the patient discuss the priorities and decide which compulsion, or set of compulsions, will be treated first (see p. 94 for the treatment of obsessions). For each selected target, the therapist asks the patient for a full account of the objects or situations that trigger the obsession and/or lead to his compulsive behaviour. A list is constructed, indicating how difficult these triggers or cues are for the patient to face. This is usually done by asking the patient to give a rating of discomfort that he estimates he will experience in each of these situations, usually on a scale of 0–100 (where 0 means 'no anxiety or discomfort' and 100 means 'extremely severe anxiety or discomfort'). An example of such a list, or hierarchy, is given in Table 7.1. Similar ratings may also be obtained for the strength of the compulsive urge, with 0 indicating 'no urge' and 100 indicating 'extremely high, irresistible urge'. If the fear of contamination is a major feature of the problem, the patient is asked to provide rating of the degree to which they feel contaminated before and after exposures (0 = not at all... 100 = totally).

Table 7.1 An example of a hierarchy of problem situations of an obsessive–compulsive patient

Items	Discomfort 0–100	Urge to wash 0–100
Using a public toilet	100	100
Touching the inside of the kitchen waste bin	95	90
Touching the toilet seat at home	80	85
Touching the outside of the kitchen waste bin	70	75
Picking up something from the kitchen floor	70	70
Shaking hands with a stranger	65	55
Using a public telephone	60	50
Touching door handles in a public place	55	45
Bumping into a stranger	55	50
Touching money given by a cashier in a supermarket	50	35

The therapist and the patient then agree on where in this list, or hierarchy, exposure should begin. Ideally, it is best to begin by tackling a point mid-way up the list, but in practice, many patients are reluctant to agree to this. Usually the starting point is the item that the patient feels willing to try despite his discomfort, provided it is not too low in terms of discomfort and compulsive urge. He is then exposed repeatedly. Exposure to several related items may be tackled together. For example, if the concern is with dirt and germs on the floor, door handles, and so on, the patient is asked to touch very thoroughly, with the therapist usually first modelling the actions, several door handles, the floor, the rim of the dust bin, and so on. The 'contamination' may then be spread to his arms and clothes by getting him to rub his hands on them. This exposure is followed by a period of response-prevention. The patient refrains from washing or engaging in any other cleaning ritual. The therapist usually stays with him during this time, providing encouragement and praise as appropriate. Physical restraint is never used in response-prevention. The therapist will be sympathetic about the patient's discomfort, and help to make it easier for him—e.g. by distraction, conversation, and so on. Early in the programme, the response-prevention period with the therapist may last for 2 hours or so; by this time, the patient's discomfort arising from the exposure, and the related compulsive urge, will normally have come down considerably. As therapy progresses, the sessions shorten to approximately 1 hour each. Sessions are held frequently in the early stages of treatment.

The details of the programme always depend on the individual patient's particular problems—no two patients are alike, and the therapist has to modify the prevailing treatment to suit each case. When the therapy is done on an out-patient basis, which happens in the vast majority of cases, some patients are given specific homework sessions to supplement the work in the clinic. If an in-patient programme is used, because of either the severity of the problems or practical difficulties in implementing therapy on an out-patient basis, attempts will be made to carry out most of the sessions away from hospital and in the home situation as soon as it is practicable.

This is a case example illustrating ERP therapy:

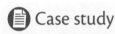# Case study

The treatment of a compulsive washer

A 22-year-old male undergraduate was referred for treatment of his intense fear of being contaminated by a dog, and the associated compulsive washing. Specifically, he feared that he might contract rabies (although he knew that the chances of this were slim) or some other serious infection. He engaged in repeated and time-consuming washing every time he felt he was contaminated; this would happen if he passed a dog or saw dog faeces on the road, if someone who had been with a dog came near him, or if he happened to touch or brush against anything to do with dogs, such as a discarded collar or a lead, or a feeding bowl. He also had engaged in a great deal of avoidance behaviour. He would cross the road to avoid having to pass a dog. He began to avoid friends and others whom he knew had dogs, and, in the end, he stopped going to classes. He would throw away any item of clothing he happened to be wearing when he went past or got anywhere near a dog. His life became very restricted as a result of this. He had no other obsessive–compulsive behaviour, except some minor checking rituals that were not causing any problems.

Initial cognitive exploration showed that the patient recognized the irrationality of his behaviour, but he did not feel totally confident that contact with dogs was safe. He was willing to accept the rationale of the therapy, and was treated with ERP, with modelling. A list of situations that caused anxiety in him was prepared on the basis of ratings of severity given by him, on a 0–100 scale. He was willing to accept exposure to the highest four items in this list. These were: touching a dog with both hands (anxiety 100); touching a bowl from which a dog had eaten (anxiety 90); touching a piece of cloth that had come in contact with a dog (anxiety 80); and walking barefoot on the ground where dogs had previously been (anxiety 75). The exposure to the first three items involved him having to touch the item very thoroughly, and then rubbing his hands on his clothes and arms. He had agreed not to wash his hands or take a bath, nor to change the affected clothes, for a period of 3 hours after each session. He had three or four treatment sessions a day. He had to keep with him, all the time, a piece of cloth that had been rubbed thoroughly on a dog in his presence, even keeping this under his pillow when he slept to ensure continuous exposure.

Despite being anxious to begin with, he cooperated well with the programme and, within a few days, was very much improved. The lower items in the original list (e.g. holding the hand of someone feeding a dog, anxiety 50) did not prove too difficult when he was later asked to do them. He began to display less avoidance behaviour, and began to move freely and use public transport.

This patient maintained his gains well. At one stage, several months later, when he noticed some signs of the problem returning, he treated himself, as he now knew what the principles of therapy were, and quickly brought the problem under control.

Therapy for other types of compulsion

The method of ERP is applicable to many types of compulsion. For checking compulsions, the patient is asked to engage in behaviour that provokes checking (e.g. using the stove, putting letters and bills into envelopes and sealing them, using electrical appliances, and so on), and then to desist from carrying out the checking. An effort is made to ensure that no reassurance is given.

In the treatment of checking, the primary components are: reducing the inflated responsibility, reducing the inflated estimates of the probability and seriousness of feared mistakes, and inhibiting the compulsion to check and re-check.

People who feel compelled repeatedly to carry out bizarre rituals are encouraged to engage in this behaviour in other, more normal, ways. For example, a patient who feels compelled to touch the four walls of a room before leaving will be given modelled exercises in the appropriate behaviour, and will keep practising the exercises until the urges decline. A patient who completely avoided his 'unsafe' number 3 felt compelled to develop bizarre methods of avoiding the number. He was encouraged to practise writing, saying, adding with the number 3, and overcame a lifelong problem within a month of regular exercising. Another patient avoided the letters A, B, and D and spent wasteful time and energy ensuring that his emails and all other communications were free of the 'unsafe' letters (during the assessment it emerged that he had been seemingly 'abandoned' for a short period as a child, and experienced a traumatic reaction, after which he developed a school phobia—hence the avoidance of the letters A, B, and D). Someone who feels compelled to ensure that all of the items on his table and in his wardrobe must be arranged in a very rigid and unchanging way will be encouraged to practise disarranging the objects repeatedly, and inhibit the urges to place them back in their precisely proper positions. These exercises are carried out daily until the urges decline.

Reduction of avoidance

The reduction of avoidance behaviour is an important component of all of the treatment programmes. Even after successful therapy focused on difficult target situations, a patient may still avoid many other situations, partly out of habit and partly because of residual worries. Patients are therefore encouraged to work systematically on overcoming any remaining unadaptive avoidance. Two case studies illustrate the reduction of avoidance.

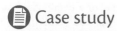 Case study

The first is a woman who avoided the 'unsafe' number 4 (see p. 54). She believed that if she did not avoid 4s, her husband would come to some harm. The avoidance encompassed most aspects of her life and dramatically restricted her functioning. The treatment concentrated on exposing her to the number 4 in numerous ways, many of them continuous. The patient was persuaded to do many activities four times, she had the number 4 painted on the walls and ceilings of her room, she carried pieces of paper with the number 4 written on them in her pockets and handbag, and so on. She practised conscientiously and achieved considerable improvement quickly.

📄 Case study

This example involves a woman who had an intense fear of developing cancer (see p. 8). She was engaging in such intensive and disabling avoidance behaviour that she had to be admitted to hospital for concentrated treatment. She avoided anything that she feared might lead her to discover signs of cancer. Her treatment programme consisted of getting her to engage in all the behaviour that she avoided, initially with supervision and help. For example, she was made regularly to look at herself in a full-length mirror, to wash and to bathe herself, to make her bed in the morning, to wash her underwear without looking away, to palpate her breasts, and so on. She had long sessions with the nurse during which she carried out these activities very thoroughly. The treatment programme led to considerable improvement within a short period of time. At the 5-year follow-up, she was still free of the problem, and leading a normal life.

Treatment of obsessions

The progress made around 30 years ago in treating compulsive behaviour, notably compulsive cleaning and compulsive checking, was not accompanied by comparable advances in dealing with obsessions. However, some progress has now been accomplished, mainly by improvements in our understanding of the nature of these unwanted, repugnant intrusive thoughts. As noted in Chapter 1, it is probable that these intrusive thoughts, which are experienced by almost everyone at one time or another, can become transformed into obsessions, if and when the person interprets them to be of great personal significance. The thoughts are interpreted by the person as being revealing, and as signifying that he is immoral, evil, dangerous, insane, or a combination of these qualities. They may also believe that the thoughts will lead to catastrophic consequences and fear that they might lose control. The thoughts are extremely distressing, and can give rise to attempts to put matters right, to neutralize, or conceal, or suppress the thoughts, and also to avoid places or people that might trigger the thoughts.

The primary aim of treatment has shifted away from the earlier methods and now focuses on the patient's interpretation of the thoughts. The therapist aims to assist the patient in making more realistic and accurate interpretations of the significance of the unwanted, intrusive thoughts. This involves an analysis of the thoughts and the meaning that the patient places on them.

The earlier methods of treatment included thought-stopping, distraction, repeated exposure to the intrusive thought (by encouraging the patient repeatedly to form the thoughts to instruction), re-shaping the intrusive images by deliberate exercise, and by discouraging the avoidance of situations in which the person was inclined to re-experience the intrusive thought. A few of these methods continue to be of some use, but are no longer the core treatment. For a period, the method known as thought-stopping was recommended as a way to help patients gain control over their unwanted intrusive thoughts. The therapist asked the patient to verbalize the obsession or thought, and, when he succeeded, the therapist shouted 'Stop'. The procedure was repeated several times until the patient was able to shout the word 'Stop' to himself whenever the unwanted thoughts intruded. This technique was of little value. Another variant involved a mildly aversive stimulus—the patient wore a rubber band on his wrist, and flicked it whenever the thoughts intruded. This was not useful.

Another approach was to get the patient repeatedly to form the thought and hold it in mind for prolonged periods, after the manner of exposure treatment. The aim of this 'habituation training' was to get the patient to become accustomed to the unwanted thought so that it gradually becomes less and less upsetting. It is seldom helpful. A similar technique is to ask the person to make a tape-recording of a description of the obsession and then listen to the audiotape repeatedly. As with the other methods of this type, the aim was to expose the patient repeatedly to the intrusions in expectation that the thoughts would eventually diminish. The value of this exposure feedback in unclear, and it does not address the patient's interpretation of the personal significance of the thoughts (e.g. 'Does it mean that I am potentially dangerous?', 'Does it mean that I wish to molest children?').

These methods are being replaced by cognitive behaviour therapy, which addresses the patient's interpretation of his intrusive thoughts. As described earlier, it has been suggested that obsessions develop when the person interprets certain of his uninvited, unwanted, and repugnant thoughts or images as being shameful and objectionable, or as being personally revealing. To take one example, 'the fact that I experience repugnant sexual thoughts and images about children means that I am a sexual predator, and potentially dangerous'. Naturally these thoughts are extremely distressing and the person tries to suppress them, to avoid places where children congregate, and to conceal the thoughts. The consequence of these decisions and actions is that the person's attempts to deal with the upsetting intrusions paradoxically enhance the importance of the thoughts. They become even more significant, and hence more frequent and more distressing.

The purpose of the therapy is to help the person develop more accurate and realistic interpretations of the personal significance of the uninvited images and thoughts. It is explained that virtually everyone experiences uninvited, unwanted images and thoughts at some time or another, even regularly, but that these intrusions are dismissed as nonsense, and of no significance. This important information is supported by the provision of lists of unwanted intrusions described by ordinary citizens. Many of these ordinary intrusions are somewhat similar in content to the patient's tormenting obsessions. A clinical problem, obsessions, arises when the person catastrophically misinterprets the personal significance of the intrusions. Characteristically, the people who are susceptible to these tormenting images and thoughts are 'of tender conscience' and high personal standards (John Bunyan and Martin Luther were among famous religious figures who suffered from obsessions).

The complete treatment of obsessions may require a considerable amount of careful therapy, depending on the severity of the problem. In mild cases, the provision of corrective information is particularly effective, and improvements can be promoted with less extensive treatment.

A 26-year-old restaurant worker complained of recurrent intrusive images and thoughts of sexually molesting children. He was distressed by these abhorrent intrusions and interpreted them as indicating that he was weird, evil, and not to be trusted. His attempts to block the images and thoughts were unsuccessful, and his only recourse was to keep away from places in which children congregate, and to avoid contact with friends who had young children. The intrusions had started in adolescence and continued with little change over the next 13 years.

During cognitive behaviour therapy it emerged that when he was 8 years of age he had been sexually abused by a neighbour over a 3-month period. The abuser told him several times that they were alike and that when the patient grew up, he too would have sexual relations with children. When the patient was 16 years old, this assertion was supported by hearing about the supposed 'cycle of abuse'; abused children grow into abusers. After detailed consideration of the patient's experiences and beliefs, his misinterpretations about himself, and, especially, the personal significance that he placed on his intrusions ('I am a paedophile'), the frequency and intensity of his obsessions declined to negligible levels. His interpretations of the intrusive images and thoughts became realistic and benign, and he discontinued his attempts to block and/or internally debate the intrusions. His avoidance behaviour extinguished. At the 12-month follow-up he remained well and completely free of the obsessions.

A 30-year-old book-keeper was tormented by recurring, horrific violent thoughts and impulses, many of them involving her parents and other members of the family. She was particularly frightened of sharp knives and took care to avoid spending time with her relatives in the family kitchen. The violent intrusions convinced her that she was potentially dangerous and becoming insane.

For several years she concealed the intrusions from other people for fear of being rejected and perhaps ending up in a long-stay hospital. After four sessions of cognitive behaviour therapy she was encouraged to tell her parents and siblings that she was receiving psychological treatment for an obsessive–compulsive disorder, and they were sympathetic and supportive. After eight sessions she was encouraged to explain to them the nature and content of her violent obsessions. They were not critical and certainly did not reject her. As before, they were sympathetic and offered their support and help. The patient's expectation that her family would share her own interpretation of the intrusions (i.e. that she was in danger of insanity and becoming violent) was flatly disconfirmed. They reassured her that she was an exceptionally kind and gentle person, trustworthy, and had never ever been violent.

Within 2 weeks of this disclosure the patient was asked if the behaviour of her family had changed. 'Now that they know about your violent thoughts, do they treat you differently? Do they seem to be frightened when you are with them in the kitchen or elsewhere? Do they look frightened when you visit them?'. In fact their behaviour towards her was unchanged, and they greeted her visits with their customary affection and pleasure. Their reactions to learning about her intrusions were important disconfirmations of the erroneous personal significance that she had attached to the intrusive images and thoughts. Her obsessions declined to very low levels and her fear of knives was extinguished. At the follow-up assessment she was free of obsessions and functioning very well.

As there is a close association between obsessions and depression, the presence or emergence of depression can lead to an increase in the intensity or frequency of the obsessions, and in these cases supplementary treatment of the depression, if necessary by anti-depressant medication, should be considered.

The main shift in emphasis that has been taking place during the past few years can be described as a movement away from helping the patient to tolerate the unwanted and uncontrollable thoughts, towards actively under-mining their occurrence by helping him to substitute more realistic and accu-rate interpretations of the significance of the intrusive thoughts themselves. This is a primarily cognitive method for dealing with a primarily cognitive problem.

Obsessional images

In some cases the obsession takes the form of mental imagery (see Table 1.3). When the patient's main problem is intrusive and repugnant images, added techniques can be useful. With some practice one can learn to manage, to manipulate one's mental images. In experiments, it has been demonstrated that most people are able to rotate, expand, shrink, rewind, and otherwise manipulate their visual images. This facility can be improved with practice. In treatment, the images can be modified in various ways. A patient whose unwanted intrusive image was of dog faeces was taught to shrink the image smaller and smaller, until it became just an innocuous dot. Another patient, who complained of distressing images of a violent scene, was trained to focus on a marginal detail of the image and 'zoom in' on this part. In this way it was possible to make this part of the image, which did not arouse discomfort, larger and larger, so that the discomfort-arousing part of the image 'overflowed' out of the image space. The image thus became less upsetting. Techniques such as these for manipulating one's unwanted images are probably effective because of the sense of control the patient gets, in successfully manipulating them. After all, one of the reasons why obsessions are a problem is that they intrude, despite resistance, and are hard to dismiss. If, therefore, the patient achieves some control over the image, that makes it less of a problem.

While these image-manipulation techniques are useful, they are not the main treatment for intrusive images. The new cognitive approach used for intrusive thoughts, described in the previous section, is equally applicable to images. Like thoughts, the images are distressing because the person attaches undue significance to them, and so helping the person to interpret them in a different way is the core treatment.

The effects of therapy

In many cases, cognitive behaviour therapy reduces the distress and difficul-ties experienced by people struggling with obsessive–compulsive disorder. The unadaptive and distressing beliefs, anxious feelings, and abnormal behaviour are reduced or even eliminated. It is important to emphasize again that the affliction of obsessive–compulsive disorder can be mild, moderate, or severe.

In mild cases, relatively minor treatment that includes authoritative information about the nature of obsessive–compulsive disorder and a few therapy sessions, supplemented by methods of self-help, can be effective. Moderately severe cases naturally require more assistance. People who have very severe obsessive–compulsive disorder almost always need concentrated treatment, and a period of hospitalization may be necessary. Improvements can be substantial; it is not correct to assume that severe cases are necessarily untreatable.

When the patient repeatedly experiences reductions in his distress and his compulsive urges, his confidence increases. A very important part of the treatment is to restore the person's damaged sense of control over the problem. The new freedom he begins to feel as his problem gradually comes under control is very rewarding. One patient said: 'I can go anywhere now. I can do so many things which I couldn't even imagine myself doing. This is wonderful.' The aim in all cases is to provide treatment that reduces the patient's distress and enables him to resume a fully functional life.

Some patients find the early stages of treatment difficult, and even drop-out, but, with practice, the treatment becomes progressively easier. Clinical researchers are currently working on refinements to make the treatment easier to complete, especially in severe cases.

The therapist needs to establish a trusting and sympathetic relationship with the patient, and to be supportive and encouraging. For moderate and severe cases, a substantial amount of therapy time may be needed: dozens of sessions rather than two or three, and they can extend over months, rather than a week or two. In-patient treatment is only recommended for those severe cases that have not benefitted sufficiently from out-patient treatment programmes.

The most important advances have been made in the treatment of contamination fears, washing, and checking compulsions, and obsessions. The treatment of compulsive hoarding, and of primary obsessional slowness has lagged behind.

Therapy for primary obsessional slowness

For those patients whose problem is primary obsessional slowness, a therapy involving pacing, prompting, and shaping is used. The patient's behaviour is paced, with repeated encouragement to shrink the time taken to complete the various self-help tasks that comprise the unadaptive pattern of extreme slowness. Time limits are agreed for selected behaviour and the patient is helped to keep to these time targets. The therapist assists by prompting the patient. Some modelling may be used as well. The therapist may demonstrate, for example, how it is possible to comb one's hair in just 2 minutes, and get the patient to do likewise. The patient is also given feedback on how well he is progressing—or not progressing—and praised for completing the tasks at, or close to, normal speed. During the early stages of treatment, patient's often ask for information about how long it should take complete these simple daily tasks—'How long should it take to put on a shoe?', 'How long should it take to tie my shoe-laces?', and so forth. They have been engaging in their exceedingly meticulous and slow behaviour for so long that they have lost sight of normal self-care, and are puzzled.

There are some exceptions, but this kind of treatment is like the problem itself, time-consuming and requires a great deal of assistance from the therapist. Some patients require hospital-based treatment initially, and after the in-patient phase, home-based therapy is also needed. These patients improve gradually, and may not retain their improvement unless further help is given by booster sessions. In exceptional cases, progress is expedited after dealing with seemingly unrelated psychological problems, such as family disputes or concealed fears. As with the problem of compulsive hoarding, significant progress in providing therapy for this disorder awaits an improved understanding of the nature and causes of primary obsessional slowness.

A 38-year-old man with chronic and severe obsessive–compulsive disorder was referred for treatment. The main feature of his disorder was excessive slowness—he took roughly 3 hours to prepare himself for work each morning. He bathed infrequently because he needed up to 5 hours to complete the process. By the time he was referred for help, he was in danger of losing his job because he was regularly late for work.

In the treatment programme, a wide range of self-care behaviour was dealt with. Only the management of brushing his teeth is cited here, as an example. Initially, he was advised and instructed on how to brush his teeth in a reasonable length of time. This produced a small impact; soon a plateau was reached beyond which no improvement took place—a typical feature with these patients. Then, the patient was asked to carry out the brushing in the presence of the therapist for a few occasions; it was clear that the slowness resulted from his wish to brush each tooth in turn, in a particular sequence, and in a meticulous manner. He was then given a demonstration of brushing teeth at normal speed, and was asked to imitate the therapist. Some improvement was obtained immediately. In the next stage of therapy, he was instructed to brush his teeth on a number of occasions during which the therapist set up a speeded-up goal and provided time checks every 30 seconds. This produced further improvement, although the patient found it difficult to break the 5-minute barrier, which was the agreed goal.

Following this approach in dealing with all of his problems, a significant overall improvement in bathing, washing, teeth-cleaning, and dressing was achieved. He steadily learned to complete his morning preparations in a reasonable time and managed to retain his job.

Other behavioural techniques

Various other behavioural treatments have also been used with obsessive–compulsive patients. One is systematic desensitization, in which the patient imagines frightening situations in a graded series of steps, while under relaxation. This was a common treatment of phobias in the early days of behaviour therapy, and nowadays is seldom used in the management of obsessive–compulsive disorders.

Contingency management is an approach that manipulates the consequences of behaviour. For example, if a patient's compulsions receive a lot of positive attention and sympathy, an attempt may be made to ensure that they cease to produce favourable results. Relatives and friends are advised accordingly and encouraged to reward adaptive alternative behaviour. Sometimes, aversive procedures are used; for example, a mild electric shock, or the use of a rubber or elastic band (see p. 95) for obsessions. These techniques are definitely not recommended.

Stress and tension tend to make obsessions and compulsions worse. For patients experiencing intense and/or persisting stress or anxiety, training in relaxation is advisable. This is a straightforward procedure in which one is instructed to relax all the major muscle groups in a series of exercises. Training in relaxation can be directly beneficial by relieving the tension and indirectly by weakening the obsessions and compulsions. Even after successful treatment, the patients may experience occasional recurrences of the obsessive–compulsive disorder problems in the wake of stressful experiences. The ability to relax oneself is a useful means of coping with periods of stress and tension. Other methods of reducing stress, such as complete stress management programmes, can be decidedly helpful.

A simple guide to relaxation is given in Appendix 1.

Problems in therapy

Effects of depression

The chances of an obsessive–compulsive patient benefiting from cognitive behaviour therapy are reduced if he is deeply depressed. In some cases, the depression even prevents the patient from participating in the treatment. These patients are best treated after their depression has been relieved by other means, usually pharmacological.

The effects of successful treatment tend to be stable, but the onset of significant depression not infrequently causes a temporary/partial return of obsessive–compulsive problems, and is dealt with by treatment of the depression and some booster sessions of cognitive behaviour therapy.

Motivation and cooperation

Some patients find the demands of a therapy, especially ERP, difficult to tolerate. This is encountered mostly when ERP is the sole or main technique to be used. This is not entirely surprising given that one is encouraged and expected repeatedly to engage the objects and situations that provoke great fear and discomfort. Patients are advised correctly that the discomfort/fear almost invariably declines fairly soon and that the programme of treatment becomes progressively easier. Therapists make an effort to persuade a reluctant patient to accept the treatment offered by answering their queries in detail and pointing out that the chances of improvement are high. A reluctant or doubting patient may be helped by the opportunity to talk with a successfully treated patient. In the end, however, the patient must decide for himself whether or not to accept therapy. Careful psychological preparation in the preliminary stages often facilitates treatment acceptance and cooperation. Recent refinements are ultimately likely to make the therapy considerably easier to tolerate.

Programmes of therapy that concentrate on, and are even confined to, cognitive methods are easy to tolerate, and there are few drop-outs or refusals, other than those that arise from practical problems, such as difficult travel arrangements. The cognitive behavioural treatment of obsessions, for example, is easily tolerable and drop-outs are not common.

Other types of psychological treatment

Hypnotherapy

Claims made by some practitioners for the effectiveness of hypnotherapy, usually involving strong suggestion to the patient while under hypnosis that he will no longer experience obsessions or compulsive urges, are not supported. There is no satisfactory evidence that hypnotherapy has much to contribute in treating these patients. Some patients and/or their families are hopeful that hypnotherapy may help, and, prior to the relatively recent development of evidence-based therapy, their search was understandable. Nowadays they are better advised to obtain therapy that is recommended by NICE.

Psychoanalysis and dynamic psychotherapy

Psychotherapy consists of psychoanalysis or its derivatives (see p. 80), usually referred to as psychodynamic therapies. These forms of therapy share the assumption that obsessions and compulsions are symptoms of underlying unconscious problems, usually psychosexual in nature. The aim of the therapy, carried out over very many sessions, sometimes extending over years, is to encourage the patient to 'free associate' (to speak openly and at length about feelings and thoughts), in order to unravel the putative hidden factors and resolve them. The relationship that develops between the patient and the therapist is considered to be very important and is said to play a part in bringing to the surface both deep-rooted conflicts and memories. The results of these types of therapy have not been satisfactory. Some patients report that prolonged psychotherapy gives them a better understanding of themselves or a better outlook on life, but the obsessive–compulsive disorder complaints seldom improve. As noted earlier, the NICE report on obsessive–compulsive disorder states that psychoanalysis is not recommended.

Group therapy

Treating patients in a group setting is sometimes undertaken for various conditions. For example, patients with upsetting social anxiety are often treated in social skills groups. There is no persuasive evidence that group therapy has any special role to play in the therapy of obsessive–compulsive patients. However, in some recent treatment programmes, patients suffering from compulsions have been successfully treated in groups; patients whose main problem is obsessions are more likely to benefit from individual treatment. Support groups for patients have been found to be of some benefit when used as an adjunct to individual therapy. Family members may also be included in the support groups. In recent years, self-help organizations have been running support groups for patients and families, and many have found these to be helpful (see Appendix 7).

Treatment of children

Cognitive behaviour therapy is effective for children, and parents/caregivers are usually involved in the treatment programme. In mild cases, a high proportion of the referrals, the provision of information and guidance often is sufficient. Moderate and severe cases require substantial treatment, and, if progress is inadequate, the addition of medication is occasionally considered.

Non-psychological treatments

Drug treatments

Pharmacological treatment is of demonstrable value in managing obsessive–compulsive disorder, and is widely used, especially in severe cases. In moderate cases, medications are often used in conjunction with psychological treatment. It is particularly useful when the patient is also suffering from significant depression. Medication has some drawbacks. Many of them produce unwanted side-effects, and coming off the medication, especially after prolonged use, can be disturbing and difficult to tolerate. For this reason, patients who are coming off the medication are strongly advised to taper it off gradually. Another problem is that some patients are given more than one such medication at a time.

A variety of medications are prescribed for obsessive–compulsive disorder usually. Anxiolytic (anxiety-reducing) benzodiazepine drugs, such as chlordiazepoxide (e.g. Librium) or diazepam (e.g. Valium). give welcome but temporary relief from the feelings of anxiety or tension, but tend to have little direct effect on the obsessions and compulsions. Phenothiazines, such as chlorpromazine (e.g. Largactil), are also occasionally prescribed but they are seldom beneficial.

Anti-depressant drugs are frequently prescribed, and varying degrees of success have been reported. In those many cases in which the obsessive–compulsive disorder is compounded by depression, treatment of the depression by drugs or psychological methods is advised. As mentioned earlier, a severely depressed obsessive–compulsive patient is unlikely to benefit from, or indeed effectively engage in, cognitive behavioural treatment. In such cases, the priority is to treat the depression. In some, the successful treatment of the depression is followed by alleviation of the obsessive–compulsive problems, and additional treatment may not be necessary. In others, reduction of the depression leaves the obsessions and compulsions weakened, but still handicapping and distressing. Psychological treatment is then advisable.

The alleviation of depression that accompanies obsessive–compulsive disorder can be achieved by standard anti-depressant medication. A list of these drugs is given in Appendix 2.

There is sound evidence that the tricyclic anti-depressant drug, clomipramine (Anafranil), can be effective in the treatment of obsessive–compulsive patients. It can be particularly efficacious in reducing depression in these patients, but is said to have a specific effect on obsessive–compulsive disorder; this claim has not yet been fully resolved. In a major study carried out in London in the 1970s, with the support of the Medical Research Council, it was observed that clomipramine did reduce both depression and obsessive–compulsive problems in a group of patients who suffered from both. However, in those patients who had little depression, clomipramine failed to produce significant improvement. The results of more recent studies do not provide a consistent picture. On balance, the evidence points to the conclusion that clomipramine is an effective treatment, especially when depression is also present; but the improvements are not always complete, and a minority of patients do not derive sufficient benefit from the drug. Recent research also suggests that the initial response to clomipramine does not provide a good prediction of the longer term effects of this medication. Patients are prone to relapse when they stop taking the drug, especially if it is stopped abruptly; tapering off under supervision is strongly recommended.

Common side-effects of clomipramine include: dryness of the mouth, constipation, dizziness, nausea, drowsiness, weight gain, and impairment of sexual functioning—particularly difficulty reaching orgasm. Clomipramine is usually started with small doses, gradually increasing to 100–250 mg/day, as necessary. Most patients take between 150 and 200 mg. The response to the medication is not immediate; it can be several weeks before any effect is seen.

Of the other anti-depressant drugs tested in recent years, encouraging results have been achieved with fluoxetine (Prozac) and fluvoxamine (Faverin, Luvox). These belong to the group of drugs called selective serotonin re-uptake inhibitors (SSRIs). Other drugs in this group include paroxetine (Seroxat, Paxil), sertraline (Lustral, Zoloft), and citalopram (Cipramil). These too have been used in the treatment of obsessive–compulsive disorder. Reports suggest that SSRIs have fewer side-effects than clomipramine. They are also safer in the event of overdoses. However, they are not free of side-effects. Possible side-effects of fluoxetine are nausea, vomiting, some insomnia, and initial increase in anxiety. Fluvoxamine can lead to headache, reduced appetite, and sweating.

Medication is commonly prescribed for severe cases of OCD, with or without psychological therapy. Often the treatment plan is to start off with medication in the expectation that when the patient is less depressed and dysfunctional, psychological treatment will follow. In cases of mild OCD, medication is not usually necessary.

The overall, long-term value of these drugs in the treatment of obsessive–compulsive disorder is still to be determined. On current evidence, long-term benefit depends on the continuation of medication. There is a distinct chance of relapse when the drug is withdrawn.

Anti-depressants used in the treatment of obsessive–compulsive disorder and the recommended dosages are given in Table 7.2.

Psychosurgery

In the past, numbers of patients with obsessive–compulsive disorder were treated with psychosurgery—i.e. surgery on the brain. Psychosurgery was originally introduced as a potential method for treating schizophrenia, and was then extended to other problems, including obsessive–compulsive disorder. The operations are used far less often now than they were a few decades ago. In fact psychosurgery is now seen as a treatment of last resort.

Table 7.2 Anti-depressants used in the treatment of obsessive–compulsive disorder

	Starting dose and increment	Usual target dose	Maximum dose
Clomipramine	10–25	100–250	250
Citalopram	20	40–60	60
Fluoxetine	20	40–60	80
Fluvoxamine	50	200	300
Paroxetine	10–20	50	60
Sertraline	50	150	225

1 Clomipramine is a tricyclic; all others are selective serotonin re-uptake inhibitors.

2 These are adult doses and are given in milligrams.

(These are based on the recommendations made by a panel of international experts as guidelines for clinical practice. Reference: March, J. S., Frances, A., Carpenter, D. and Kahn, D. A. (1997). Treatment of obsessive–compulsive disorder (Expert Consensus Guideline Series). *Journal of Clinical Psychiatry*, **58** (Supplement 4).

It is an invasive and drastic form of treatment, although the techniques used are now much more refined than they were, and therefore have fewer side-effects than in the early days. Moderate effects have been claimed in some patients with chronic intractable obsessions or compulsions, but in many others the results of psychosurgery have been unsatisfactory. The NICE report on OCD states that psychosurgery is not recommended.

Electroconvulsive therapy (ECT)

Occasionally, severe cases of obsessive–compulsive are treated with ECT (electric shock therapy). In this procedure, convulsions are induced by passing a small electric current through the brain from electrodes applied to the head, while the patient is under the effects of an anaesthetic and muscle relaxant. It is painless, and the patient retains no memory of the procedure. Modern improvements have made the treatment more tolerable.

There is no evidence that ECT has any directly beneficial effects on obsessive–compulsive disorder, as such, but it can be indirectly beneficial if it reduces coexisting depression. In severe cases of obsessive–compulsive disorder, ECT is considered if the patient is deeply depressed and has received little or no benefit from other treatments, including a full range of medications.

8

Assessment, diagnosis, and evaluation

➔ Key points

◆ The assessment of obsessive–compulsive disorders includes comprehensive interviews, psychological tests, and behavioural observations.

◆ The assessments are necessary for diagnosis, planning of treatment, and evaluation of progress.

◆ There are no laboratory tests for obsessive–compulsive disorder.

◆ The assessment includes a determination of the severity of the problem.

◆ The three categories—mild, moderate, or severe—are based on the amount of distress the patient is experiencing and the extent to which his life is compromised by the disorder.

Clinical assessments are carried for three reasons:

◆ diagnosis;

◆ planning of treatment;

◆ evaluating the effects of treatment.

The methods used for these purposes overlap to some extent but are distinctive. Naturally, if the diagnostic assessment shows that the person does not have an obsessive–compulsive disorder there is no need for further assessments.

Diagnosis

The first step is to determine if the person has the disorder. The initial and essential part of the diagnostic process is a detailed interview. This is supplemented by psychological tests that consist of questionnaires and behavioural avoidance tests.

The assessor—psychologist, doctor, or psychiatrist—will look for particular features that are distinctive of the disorder, and also consider related possibilities. It is necessary to decide whether or not the person has an obsessive–compulsive disorder and then whether he also other problems, such as depression. The criteria used in the diagnosis are listed in Table 1.2. In most cases, the diagnosis is fairly straightforward, but some problems can be encountered if the person has associated psychological problems.

Outside of the health professions, obsessive–compulsive disorders are not widely understood and, as mentioned earlier, there is a tendency for it to be over-diagnosed. In clinical practice, a number of people referred for the assessment of this disorder prove to have some other disorder, or none at all. Importantly, not all troublesome worries are obsessions, and not all types of repetitive behaviour are compulsions. It is essential to complete a comprehensive clinical assessment in determining whether or not the person has an obsessive–compulsive disorder.

A majority of people with obsessive–compulsive disorder have concurrent depression or have had episodes of depression in the past. It is not uncommon for the obsessive–compulsive disorder to be accompanied by other disorders, such as social phobia, which may complicate the diagnosis, and the diagnostician may have to decide which disorder is primary, and determine if there is a significant relationship between the obsessive–compulsive disorder and the associated diagnosis.

Once the diagnosis is established, a more detailed assessment is undertaken. The main purpose of this is to gather information for devising a treatment programme. As these patients are best treated by cognitive behaviour therapy, detailed information about the patient's cognitions is needed in order to plan effective treatment. The assessment also provides a baseline against which the effects of the treatment can be gauged. Assessment is necessary to evaluate the immediate and continuing effects of the treatment. Hence, the post-treatment assessments are likely to be repeated, usually at 6 months and again at 12 months after the completion of treatment.

There are no laboratory tests for obsessive–compulsive disorder.

How is assessment done?

The main techniques of assessment used by therapists are summarized in the following paragraphs.

Interview with the patient

The main part of the assessment is a comprehensive interview. This may take 2 or 3 hours, spread over more than one session. The patient will be asked for full details of the problems, including how they affect work, relationships, and social life. Questions will be asked about how and when it all started and what the course of the disorder has been, including fluctuations in severity, relationship to stressful events, and so on. As for the problems themselves, close inquiry will be made about each presenting problem, and the person's thoughts about them.

For obsessions, these inquiries will focus, among others, on the following aspects:

◆ What is the content of the obsession?

◆ What form (thought, image, or impulse, or a combination) does it take?

◆ Is it triggered by any event or object?

◆ How long does it last when it comes?

◆ How much anxiety or discomfort does it lead to?

◆ How do you try to get rid of it?

◆ Does it lead to a compulsion?

◆ What is the personal significance of the obsession?

◆ Is it revealing of anything important to you?

◆ Do you conceal them from other people, and if so, why?

◆ Do you think that the obsessions may lead to dangerous or objectionable behaviour?

◆ Do you ever think that the obsessions mean that you are weird?

- If the person describes an extreme fear of contamination:

  - What places, items, and people provoke the feelings?

  - What do you fear the contamination will lead to?

  - How and when did the fear arise?

  - Does it interfere with your life?

  - Does it lead to the avoidance of people, places, and activities? How do you attempt to deal with the feelings?

For compulsions, the following questions will probably be asked:

- What is the nature of the compulsive behaviour?

- What events or objects lead to the urge to carry out the compulsive behaviour?

- How strong is the urge?

- How frequently does it occur?

- Is it observable behaviour or carried out internally, or both?

- How long does it take to carry out the compulsion?

- Is it performed a specific number of times?

- What is the significance of that number?

- How much do you resist the urge?

- What happens if the compulsive behaviour is interrupted?

- What do you think or believe will happen if you do not carry out the compulsion?

- Do you feel a special responsibility to prevent such consequences by personally carrying out the ritual?

Ordinarily, all of the aspects of obsessive–compulsive phenomena summarized in Table 1.3 will be gone into. The therapist will also explore the relationship between the problems and mood, and usually ask about possible depression, present or past.

In addition to the conventional diagnostic interviews used by most clinicians, a number of specialized methods have been developed for purposes of clinical research and/or in clinics that provide specialist treatment for obsessive–compulsive disorder. These specialized interviews are called 'structured' because the diagnostician follows a carefully constructed, strict manual, which ensures that all of the questions are asked, in exactly the same manner and sequence for every patient, by every interviewer. The structured interview schedules used in assessing obsessive–compulsive disorder range from a broad scale, which assesses mental health in general (the SCID, Structured Clinical Interview), to a scale that focuses exclusively on anxiety disorders (the ADIS, Anxiety Disorders Interview Schedule), and finally to the most specific scale, which provides assessments of the nature and severity of the obsessive–compulsive disorder (the Y-BOCS, Yale-Brown Obsessive–Compulsive Scale). As the scales become more specialized, they enable the clinician (or research worker) to increase the 'magnification of the microscope'.

Self-ratings

Most therapists will ask the patient to rate the discomfort and the urge to ritualize on a numerical scale (see p. 115). Some use a 0–10 scale, others prefer a 0–8 scale, while still others use a 0–100 scale. The last mentioned is easy for the patient to use and is recommended by many. Sometimes, especially with children, a visual analogue scale is used instead. This is simply a straight line, usually 100 mm in length, one end of which indicates the highest possible level of what is being measured (such as extremely high discomfort), and the other the absence of it (e.g. no discomfort at all). The patient indicates where, on this line, his response lies. The therapist can convert this into a numerical score by simply measuring the distance from the 'low' end to the place marked by the patient, as in Fig. 8.1.

In preparation for therapy, various situations (e.g. using a public telephone or leaving the house without checking gas taps) that are relevant to the patient's problems will be listed, with ratings of discomfort and of compulsive urge. For each main problem, a separate list or hierarchy may be prepared. An example of such a list is given in Table 7.1.

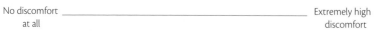

No discomfort _____ Extremely high
at all   discomfort

Fig. 8.1 A visual analogue scale sometimes used for rating discomfort.

Interviewing others

Interviewing a family member or other key informant is also part of the assessment, whenever possible. Some aspects of the patient's problems are often more clearly described by a family member than by the patient himself. For example, problems and stresses caused by the patient's behaviour and the demands on the family may be minimized in the patient's own account. Sometimes a patient has no realistic idea of the extent of his own disability, and information from the family or other informants will be valuable. Occasionally, information may be sought from work colleagues or employers. Contact with family and employers is made only with the patient's informed and written consent.

Behavioural tests and direct observation

Sometimes a therapist may carry out one or more behavioural test with the patient. For example, a patient with contamination fears about dirt and germs on door handles, public telephones, and so on, may be asked to touch a door handle during the interview session. The patient's reaction, his attempts to avoid this, and his ratings of the discomfort felt while carrying out the action are all important information for the therapist. Behavioural tests may also be carried out at home or, less frequently, at work. Direct observation at home or at work may also be undertaken. For example, a man whose obsessional slowness began to affect his efficiency at work was observed by the therapist for a set period of time, with prior agreement.

Record-keeping by the patient

It is common for a therapist to ask the patient to keep a daily record of his problem behaviour for a week or two prior to starting therapy, as a baseline measure. It may be continued during therapy as a way of monitoring progress. The record can either be an open-ended account, in which the patient writes in detail what happens, or, more commonly, a record using a structured format provided by the therapist. An example of a structured record form is given in Fig. 8.2 and a completed record form in Fig. 8.3. As can be seen, the record focuses on selected target problems, which are briefly recorded. Such structured records are easier to use and much more amenable to analysis than open-ended accounts. Another problem with open-ended accounts is that many obsessive–compulsive patients write pages and pages of detail. One patient who was asked to keep a written record of his daily problems for a week produced a sheaf of over a hundred pages in very small, neat handwriting.

Date   Target[1]

Time	Frequency[2]	Highest discomfort[3]	Highest compulsive urge[4]	Details and comments[5]
Before 7 a.m.				
7–10 a.m.				
10 a.m.– 1 p.m.				
1–4 p.m.				
4–7 p.m.				
7–10 p.m.				
After 10 p.m.				

1   The particular obsession or compulsion monitored.
2   How many times it happened in each time period.
3, 4   Rated on a 0–100 scale; give the highest felt during the time period.
5   Details of what happened; when, where, what was the trigger, how long taken,
      number of repetitions, and so on, of the <u>worst</u> episode.

Fig. 8.2 An example of a daily record sheet, blank.

Date: *27 September*   Target:[1] *Hand-washing*

Time	Frequency[2]	Highest discomfort[3]	Highest compulsive urge[4]	Details and comments[5]
Before 7 a.m.	2	70	70	*After using toilet. Washed hands with soap, 3 min.*
7–10 a.m.	3	80	85	*After journey to work by bus. Felt quite dirty. Washed with soap, 4 min.*
10 a.m.– 1 p.m.	0			*In office all the time.*
1–4 p.m.	2	60	60	*After going to the toilet. Washed with soap, 3 min.*
4–7 p.m.	3	85	90	*Felt very dirty after return journey in crowded bus. Washed with soap, 5 min.*
7–10 p.m.	1	40	45	*Before supper. Washed without soap, 1 min.*
After 10 p.m.	2	70	75	*After cleaning toilet. Washed with soap also arms, 5 min.*

1   The particular obsession or compulsion monitored.
2   How many times it happened in each time period.
3, 4   Rated on a 0–100 scale; give the highest felt during the time period.
5   Details of what happened; when, where, what was the trigger, how long taken, number of
      repetitions, and so on, of the <u>worst</u> episode.

Fig. 8.3 An example of a daily record sheet, completed.

Questionnaires and inventories

Standard questionnaires and similar instruments are also used in assessment. These have the advantage of covering a range of difficulties and producing a numerical summary score. These are, however, not used as a substitute for interview, but as an additional measure. Checklists, questionnaires, and inventories are often used in this way, and are helpful for planning treatment and assessing progress after treatment, and at follow-up assessments. They are commonly used in research projects. Some patients relish them but others find it difficult to respond to questionnaire items, and spend hours agonizing over the precise accuracy of their replies. If the completion of the questionnaires takes excessive time or is upsetting, they can be omitted or delayed.

Some commonly used instruments are described below.

The Maudsley Obsessional–Compulsive Inventory

A widely use self-report instrument for obsessive–compulsive patients is the Maudsley Obsessional–Compulsive Inventory (MOCI), which was developed in the 1970s at the Maudsley Hospital in London. The MOCI consists of 30 items. The patient has to choose either 'true' or 'false' for each item. The inventory yields an overall obsessive–compulsive symptom score, and, in addition, separate sub-scores for checking, washing, and cleaning, slowness and repetitiveness, and doubting and conscientiousness.

These are a few items from the MOCI:

◆ I avoid using public telephones because of possible contamination.

◆ I use only an average amount of soap.

◆ Some numbers are extremely unlucky.

◆ I do not tend to check things more than once.

◆ One of my major problems is that I pay too much attention to detail.

The full inventory and the scoring key are reproduced in Appendix 3 and Appendix 4, respectively.

The MOCI is easy to use, and has been shown to be a useful part of assessment. It has been established as a standard instrument in several countries. However, it is now out of date, and has been replaced by an expanded version, the Vancouver Obsessional Compulsive Inventory (VOCI).

The Compulsive-Activity Checklist

This instrument is used both for self-rating by the patient and for ratings by the therapist. The Compulsive-Activity Checklist (CAC) lists 39 specific activities (e.g. having a bath or shower, brushing teeth, cleaning the house, switching lights and taps on or off, touching door handles, filling in forms, eating in restaurants, and throwing things away). Each activity is rated on a 4-point scale of severity, from 0 (no problems with the activity) to 3 (unable to complete or attempt the activity). The total score is obtained by adding the scores of the individual items. The total score, however, is less important than the range of activities that present problems in the patient's life, and the identification of those activities that are impossible or extremely difficult to complete.

The CAC was developed in the 1970s at the Maudsley Hospital in London. It is used in many clinics and hospitals.

The Padua Inventory

The Padua Inventory (PI) was developed by Ezio Sanavio in Italy. It has 60 items, scored from 0 (not at all disturbing) to 4 (very much disturbing). Thus the range of scores is from 0 to 240. The PI has recently been used and standardized in some other countries as well.

Here are some items of the PI:

- I feel my hands are dirty when I touch money.

- I wash my hands more often and longer than necessary.

- Before going to sleep I have to do certain things in a certain order.

- I sometimes have an impulse to hurt defenceless children or animals.

- When I hear about a disaster, I think it is somehow my fault.

The Obsessive–Compulsive Inventory

The Obsessive–Compulsive Inventory (OCI) was developed a few years ago. It consists of 42 items, comprising seven sub-scales: washing, checking, doubting, ordering, obsessing, hoarding, and mental neutralization. For each item, a 5-point rating scale is used for frequency and distress over the past month.

The Yale-Brown Obsessive–Compulsive Scale

The Yale-Brown Obsessive–Compulsive Scale (Y-BOCS), which was mentioned earlier, is a widely used interview schedule that covers the main types of obsessions and compulsions, and enables the therapist to estimate the severity of the disorder. A brief self-report version has also been developed, and can be used in clinical assessment. The Y-BOCS is limited because various aspects of obsessive–compulsive disorder are not covered, many replies are collected but not scored, there are no questions about the person's cognitions or scoreable questions about avoidance, and problems of interpretation arise. It is useful in diagnosis but needs to be supplemented by other measures, and its value in assessing the progress of psychological treatment is limited.

Other scales

The Symmetry, Ordering and Arranging Questionnaire (SOAQ), a scale for assessing compulsive ordering and related behaviour, is available, and is reproduced in Appendix 5.

Instruments for assessing related problems

The therapist may also use other inventories to measure depression, anxiety, phobias, and so on, as deemed relevant for a full assessment. As noted, depression often is associated with obsessions and compulsions, and many therapists include it in routine assessment. The most widely used screening instrument for assessing depression is the Beck Depression Inventory (BDI). Developed by Dr Aaron T. Beck and his colleagues, it comprises 21 items covering areas such as mood, self-esteem, sleep, appetite, feelings of guilt, sex drive, suicidal ideas, and so on. For each item, the patient is asked to indicate whether he has experienced the affect or change in behaviour and, if so, to what degree. Scores of 0–3 are obtained for each item, yielding a possible maximum of 63. Scores above 10 are taken as showing the presence of mild depression, scores above 16 indicating moderate depression, and scores above 25 indicating severe depression. These cut-off points are not absolute and are only used as a rough guide.

For assessing general anxiety, there are several instruments, including the Beck Anxiety Inventory, which, like the BDI, has 21 items each scored from 0 to 3. The total score is 63.

Psychophysiological assessment

Psychophysiological measures are sometimes undertaken with obsessive–compulsive patients. The activity of the autonomic nervous system, especially heart rate and skin conductance, may be measured under various conditions—e.g. while exposed to triggers, and after carrying out a compulsive ritual. While such measures are valuable for research, their usefulness in routine clinical assessment is limited. In most clinical settings these recordings are not used.

Assessment for evaluating therapy

In a systematic approach, the patient will be assessed in some or all of the above ways at several points in time: before treatment begins, after a period of therapy, at the end of therapy, and at follow-up, usually 6 and 12 months later. In this way, the patient's progress can be ascertained formally and methodically. The numerical scores, in particular, help to highlight the changes in the patient. For example, assuming successful therapy, a patient's whose MOCI score was 21 at initial assessment may have a score of 7 at the 6-month follow-up. A situation that evoked a discomfort level of 90 (on a 0–100 scale) before therapy may not provoke more than 10 after therapy. The frequency of handwashing, which was 12 times a day on average before therapy, may now be only twice per day.

The Y-BOCS is often used for assessing the progress of psychological therapy but it was not designed for that purpose and has the limitations mentioned above.

Severe, mild, or moderate?

In the course of reaching a diagnosis, a determination is made about the severity of the disorder. The factors that are taken into account include:

◆ The frequency of the problem behaviour.

◆ The intensity of the problem behaviour.

◆ The distress caused by or associated with the problem.

◆ The nature and extent of associated avoidance behaviour.

◆ The degree to which the problem interrupts or prevents preferable activities.

◆ The extent to which the problem disturbs satisfactory personal relationships.

- The extent to which the problem interferes with or prevents social life.

- The nature and extent of family disruptions that arise from the problem.

- The extent to which the problem interferes with or prevents a working life.

- The extent to which the person is housebound.

- The extent to which the person 'lives at night' and sleeps long and late during the day.

- The extent to which the problem interferes with or prevents travel.

- The duration of the problem.

- Responses to previous treatments.

- The extent to which the person has an 'obsessional life-style', a life dominated by the obsessive–compulsive disorder.

This information is gathered during the clinical interview, and whenever possible is supplemented by an (less extensive) interview with a family member or close friend. It is advisable to collect information from specialized psychological tests, such as the Vancouver Obsessive–Compulsive Inventory, or similar, and from the standardized interview for obsessive–compulsive disorders (Y-BOCS), because it provides information about severity, despite its limitations.

The severity of the disorder is affected by the presence/absence of associated disorders (referred to as 'co-morbidity'). In obsessive–compulsive disorders, anxiety is invariably present and a high proportion of patients have co-morbid depression. In the absence of other disorders, it is likely that the obsessive–compulsive disorder will fall into the mild to moderate category.

9

Obsessive–compulsive disorders in children

> ## ➡ Key points
>
> ◆ Obsessive–compulsive disorders do occur in children.
>
> ◆ The symptoms and features of the disorder resemble those observed in adults.
>
> ◆ The incidence is low.
>
> ◆ A majority of the children who manifest symptoms of the disorder 'grow out of it'.
>
> ◆ Approximately 10% who continue to suffer from the disorder into adulthood tend to fall into the severe category.
>
> ◆ The psychological treatment that is used to treat adults, cognitive behaviour therapy, is also effective in the treatment of children but is modified to make it understandable and acceptable to children.
>
> ◆ The diagnostic process can be complicated by the tendency of affected children to minimize the problem.
>
> ◆ In the assessment of the child's problems it is essential to collect a good deal of information from the parents and teachers.

Obsessive–compulsive disorders can occur in childhood. It is estimated that between 0.5 and 2% of children and adolescents can be affected by the disorder. In most respects, the symptoms and features resemble those seen in adults. It usually takes the form of repetitive, compulsive behaviour, and, as with adults, compulsive cleaning and compulsive checking are the most common manifestations. The compulsion to arrange objects and order tasks inflexibly, and the drive for symmetry, are more frequently seen in children than in adults. The compulsion to count, and the compulsion to ask others to repeat utterances and actions, are common in obsessive–compulsive children. Very often the compulsive behaviour, the checking, cleaning, or ordering, is carried out in an attempt to prevent or ward off harm. The child has an inflated fear of harm coming to parents, relatives, friends, or self, and tries to protect people by carrying out the compulsive activities. In some, however, the compulsive behaviour has no such basis; instead, the compulsion is driven by a sense that 'it is not right' or 'it does not feel right'.

> An 8-year-old girl spent long hours each day arranging and ordering all of her possessions, books, and clothes in a fixed pattern, as a means of preventing her mother from dying. The family had been involved in a motor vehicle accident that severely injured the patient's mother, leaving her bleeding and semi-conscious. Prior to the accident, the child had been 'nervous' and this quality was greatly increased after the accident. She was easily startled, clinging, and tearful, and her sleep was disturbed. After the accident, she changed from a neat and tidy child into a compulsive checker with a drive to keep her possessions in a strict, inflexible order. When this overwhelming need to protect her mother and other relatives became evident she was reassured in a few sessions, accompanied by her parents, that the family was in no particular danger and that her father and mother were reliable, strong, and responsible. As the child's feelings that she bore special responsibility for protecting the family subsided, the compulsions faded out.

Differences from superstitions

Some of the beliefs and repetitive actions resemble superstitions. Unlike superstitious behaviour, however, the beliefs and rituals noted in childhood obsessive–compulsive disorder are concerned exclusively with negative thoughts, with threats of harm, which then lead to a need to carry out protective actions. Unlike superstitions, the troubling ideas in obsessive–compulsive disorder always involve emotions, especially sadness and fear, and are not regarded by the child as being the same as superstitions. Many superstitious beliefs, and the associated actions, are positive, and are attempts to bring good luck, but OCD thoughts and actions are emotional, intense, one-sided, and entirely concerned with the possibility of misfortune; they are always negative. Obsessive–compulsive disorder is not easily open to rational analysis and to rational change.

Table 9.1 Comparison of obsessive–compulsive problems and superstitions in children

Obsessive–compulsive problems	Superstitious beliefs and behaviour
Compulsions are driven, repetitive, intense behaviour, which at times the child will attempt to resist and which usually are recognized by him as being excessive. Typical examples include repetitive, compulsive washing to remove dirt or germs. Failure to complete the compulsion, especially if it is interrupted, can cause distress. The compulsions and their driving force are personal to the affected child and not shared by other children or members of the family.	Concerned with good and bad luck, they are seldom resisted by the child, and rarely cause distress. Superstitions are irrational or magical beliefs that are shared by other children or adults. Unlike obsessions, they are not unique and personal.

In some instances, it is difficult to distinguish between obsessive–compulsive ideas and behaviour, and superstitious beliefs and behaviour. As Table 9.1 illustrates, there are, however, some simple tests that can be applied in trying to make the distinction between superstitious beliefs and habits, and obsessive–compulsive problems.

Features of childhood obsessive–compulsive disorder

The unwanted, intrusive, repugnant, and recurrent thoughts (obsessions) that affect many adult patients are seldom described by children. Two of the three major themes of adult obsessions, those that involve blasphemy and/or unacceptable sexual ideas, are rarely encountered. Fears of losing control and unwillingly harming people occasionally emerge in adolescence. The cognitive biases described on p. 7 are seldom evident in children with obsessive–compulsive disorder.

As with adults, there is an association between obsessive–compulsive disorder and depression in children. The depression is as likely to follow the obsessive–compulsive disorder as to precede it. In cases of childhood obsessive–compulsive disorder, a slight elevation of psychological problems is found in members of the family. Between 10 and 20% of parents are likely to have experienced some form of anxiety disorder or mood disorder. The gender distribution is different from that in adult patients. Among children there is a male to female ratio of 3:2. The age of onset appears to be earlier for boys than for girls. Roughly half of children with obsessive–compulsive disorder also have significant social fears, and a significant minority have eating problems. Up to a third of them are excessively perfectionistic.

In the continuous study of the development of all 1037 children born in Dunedin, New Zealand in 1972, it was found that 182 of them had at least one symptom of obsessive–compulsive disorder by the age of 11. Reassuringly, only 18 still had any obsessive–compulsive disorder symptoms by the age of 21; that is, 90% of the participants had lost their symptoms. As few of the children had received formal treatment, the findings suggest that most young children do 'grow out of it'. However, the prospects can be troubling for those children who do not improve spontaneously during childhood. Without treatment, obsessive–compulsive disorder can become a chronic problem, and in severe cases is incapacitating. One-third of adult cases report that their obsessive–compulsive disorder began in some form or other during childhood. In the Dunedin study, those who developed severe obsessive–compulsive disorder showed a history of behavioural problems of various kinds during childhood. As with adult obsessive–compulsive disorder, the effect on the child's life can be serious. It can lead to social isolation, disruption of education, family conflicts, and a distressing brew of fear, sadness, and frustration.

Signs of the disorder

What are the signs of obsessive–compulsive disorder in children? The most obvious signs of an obsessive–compulsive problem in a child are behavioural. If the child is seen to engage in intense repetitive checking, cleaning, or ordering for lengthy periods of time, and to do so in a way that interferes with, or prevents, ordinary activities such as studying, dressing, eating, bathing, and so on, one needs to take notice. If this intense and repetitive behaviour is rigid and resistant to change, it may signal an obsessive–compulsive disorder, particularly if the child reacts emotionally to interruptions or interference with the activities (such as interfering with the fixed inflexible patterning and arranging of their possessions). More often than not, the child will be unable to explain the reason for the behaviour and may resort to saying, 'I must do it *right*', or 'I have to keep doing it until it feels *right*'. Accompanying signs may be depression and/or social withdrawal or isolation. As the compulsions can demand a great deal of time, the child may leave other tasks undone and appear to be very slow to complete tasks. In cases in which perfectionism is prominent, the child devotes meticulous attention to tasks, especially studying, and may have to produce numerous copies of assignments before they are satisfied. They show inflexibility and often are late, with a strong tendency to procrastinate. They resist suggestions that their perfectionistic behaviour is excessive and self-defeating, and resist the adoption of more flexible aims and habits.

Some case studies are presented below.

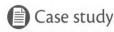 # Case study

A 14-year-old boy complained of a variety of troubling obsessions, inde-cisiveness, repeated checking, and washing his hands up to 30 times per day. Many of his obsessions concerned harm coming to others (e.g. being involved in a car accident) and violent images of a catastrophic nature. In response to the obsessions, he felt compelled to wash his hands repeatedly. In addition, he felt driven to repeat whatever action he had been engaged in when the obsession occurred (e.g. repeatedly packing his school bag, repeatedly putting on his shoes). At school he had to re-read book chap-ters four times, and repeatedly check and correct all of his written work (he had used so much correcting fluid that his teacher was obliged to ban it completely). The tedium and stress involved in trying to get his home-work 'just right' was so great that he began avoiding it totally. He ate his food in a ritual manner, and strictly avoided sharing food with anyone else because of his fears of harm.

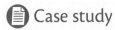 # Case study

A 12-year-old-girl was frightened of a range of objects, which she felt might be dangerously contaminated, and took care to avoid any house-hold items that contained warnings on the label, sticky substances, urine on lavatory seats, and so on. She was also fearful of raw meat and a vari-ety of possible sources of germs. The underlying fear was that harm might come to her, other people, or pets. She also complained of obsessional impulses that she might cause harm, express obscenities, or steal. She attempted to control the distress caused by these fears and obsessions by widespread avoidance, and by compulsive cleaning and checking activi-ties. Her checking was taking up to 3 hours per day, and the cleaning 2 hours per day. In addition, she repeatedly sought reassurance from her parents that they were safe.

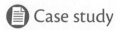 Case study

Glynis was an intensely preoccupied and serious child from an early age. At the age of 7 it became apparent to her parents that she was widely fearful and constantly dreaded that 'something horrible will happen to me'. In order to protect herself from the anticipated but vague catastrophe, she became exceedingly cautious and inflexible. She had to prepare and wear her limited range of clothes in a carefully prescribed order and fashion, rarely strayed from her 'safe' routes, ate in a slow and inflexible manner, spent 2 hours per day showering, and so on.

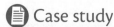 Case study

Nine-year-old Michael developed a serious fear of germs, washed a lot, and ate a very narrow range of foods that had to be 'hygienically' prepared (he inspected the entire cutlery meticulously). He insisted on precision in all matters, large and small, and was easily provoked to anger if his family failed to comply with his needs and fears.

Diagnosis and assessment

It is important to bear in mind that the child rarely complains of compulsions or obsession. Even when parents, friends, and teachers see signs of significant obsessive–compulsive disorder problems, the affected child is likely to minimize or even deny the problem. Naturally this can obscure the identification of childhood obsessive–compulsive disorder. In order to tackle this problem of differing reports, Professor R. Shafran and her colleagues developed a self-report scale, the Children's Obsessive–Compulsive Inventory (Ch-OCI), to be filled in by the child and a version for the parent to fill in on the child's behalf.

The Ch-OCI consists of two parts. The first deals with compulsive behaviour (called 'habits' in the instrument). There are 10 items, for example:

♦ I spend a lot of time every day checking things over and over again.

♦ I always count, even when doing ordinary things.

The second part is about obsessions (called 'thoughts' in the instrument). Again there are 10 items, for example:

◆ I often have bad thoughts that make me feel like a terrible person.

◆ I can't stop upsetting myself about death going round in my head, over and over again.

For each part, an additional section enquires about the extent of the most upsetting habits, and the most prominent thoughts.

The parents' version of the Ch-OCI is exactly the same except that the parent is asked to fill it in to reflect the habits/thoughts of their son or daughter.

The Ch-OCI is reproduced in Appendix 6.

Unlike the standard clinical diagnostic interviews for childhood obsessive–compulsive disorder, which typically yield a gap between the reports given by the child and the parent, the Ch-OCI tends to produce comparable results for the child and parent. However, the scale is merely a supplement to the standard diagnostic interview techniques and the children's version of the Yale scale for measuring obsessive–compulsive disorder (see p. 118). The children's version of the Yale interview schedule (CY-BOCS) is an extension of the adult version (Y-BOCS). The use of the CY-BOCS is generally preceded by the standardized interview schedule, the child and the parent version of the Diagnostic Interview Schedule (DISC), which tests for a range of psychological and psychiatric problems including depression.

If a child displays intense inflexible compulsive behaviour of the type set out above, and if there are accompanying signs, then the possibility of obsessive–compulsive disorder is worth considering. In preparing for a medical/psychological opinion, completion of the Ch-OCI may be a useful preliminary step.

In addition to the standardized interviews and formal tests that comprise the assessment of obsessive–compulsive disorder in children, it is advisable to have a period of observation of the child's behaviour, especially if it is thought that the child is underplaying the difficulties. As mentioned, in many instances the obsessive–compulsive disorder is accompanied by other problems, such as social anxiety and depressed mood. Some children with obsessive–compulsive disorder are extremely demanding and controlling, and tend to become upset and angry when their compulsions are interrupted or blocked by others. Some severely affected children try to control the entire family in an attempt to deal with their anxiety and the associated compulsive behaviour.

Some diagnostic problems

Tourette syndrome

Diagnostic problems sometimes arise from confusion between the purposeful, meaningful, intentional compulsive behaviour, such as cleaning and checking, and repetitive but purposeless twitches or tics. In some cases of severe tic disorders, such as Tourette syndrome (see pp. 32–33), compulsive behaviour is evident. Among the majority of children with obsessive–compulsive disorder, the occurrence of major and disruptive tics is not common. However, some children with obsessive–compulsive disorder do have Tourette syndrome, and a few differences have been reported between obsessive–compulsive children who also have Tourette syndrome and those who do not. Those with Tourette syndrome have more touching, counting, and blinking compulsions, and fewer cleaning compulsions, than those who do not have Tourette syndrome.

Autism

Obsessive–compulsive problems in children also need to be distinguished from childhood autism, also called 'autistic disorder'. Some of the clinical features of autism superficially resemble symptoms of obsessive–compulsive disorder. These include: a strict adherence to rigid routines or rituals, repetitive motor behaviour (such as specific movements of hands or whole body movements), and preoccupation with details of things, which to others appear irrelevant or unimportant. Autistic children dislike change, and tend to maintain 'sameness'. They do not easily respond to attempts to alter their 'habits'.

While these factors seem to overlap with some of the symptoms of childhood obsessive–compulsive disorder, autistic children also have other, prominent deficits. These include impairment of social interactions, including, in many cases, an inability to respond to others' emotions, and difficulties or abnormalities in communication. These deficits are not part of obsessive–compulsive problems in children.

Autism is essentially what child psychologists and psychiatrists call a developmental disorder, i.e. it is a disorder that first appears in infancy or early childhood. In the case of autism, diagnostic criteria stipulate that delays or abnormal functioning in social interaction, language, or symbolic/imaginative play are detected before the age of 3.

Treatment

The literature on the treatment of children with obsessive–compulsive disorder is limited, largely because of the relatively small number of cases reported. The best treatment is the same kind of psychological therapy used with adult patients—especially a combination of exposure and response-prevention for those who engage in observable compulsions. The specifically cognitive elements that are commonly used in the treatment of adults (see Chapter 7) have limited relevance in the treatment of children, particularly the younger ones. Medication may play a useful role, especially if the child is depressed. Parents are involved in the treatment and given advice and help on how to deal with the child's problem behaviour, especially his demands for things to be done in a certain way, or repeated requests for reassurance.

As mentioned earlier, there are no golden rules for family members to follow; each child and each family is unique. In general, the parents are advised to act in a comforting but firm manner. In many instances some minor compromises are agreed, but as far as possible parents should refrain from getting involved in the child's compulsions and rituals. Once a problem has been recognized parents should seek professional advice, and, if treatment is recommended, they should arrange this without delay.

Some parents also need help with basic child management techniques. Work with the family is an important part of therapy since family members may need a good deal of help and support. Formal family therapy may be undertaken in addition to the specific behavioural treatment; indeed, some therapists consider this to be an integral part of therapy. The child's school and the teachers are sometimes involved in the treatment programme in order to ensure consistency in the way adults respond to the child's behaviour. Mild cases tend to respond very well to treatment. In some cases, the severity of the problem makes a period in hospital necessary. It is well to bear in mind that the large majority of children who display some features of obsessive–compulsive disorder do 'grow out of it'.

Much research on childhood obsessive–compulsive problems is being carried out, and there is every reason to expect significant advances in treatment in the future.

10

Some practical advice

Key points

- Obsessive–compulsive disorders are treatable.

- If you are concerned that you or a relative might have the disorder, there are a few key questions that can guide you, and some elementary tests are provided in the Appendices.

- There are several non-profit self-help groups that provide valuable information and advice.

- It is advisable to consult your family doctor, who might recommend that you seek a full investigation of the problem.

- A comprehensive assessment, along the lines described in Chapter 8, is recommended.

Is there a problem?

Many people experience mild obsessions and compulsions occasionally, but for the great majority of them these are not significant. The person concerned is not troubled or concerned about them, and neither seeks nor wants assistance. There is nothing faulty or abnormal in your behaviour if you check your gas cooker twice before you leave home every morning, or are fastidious about cleanliness, or strive always to be absolutely punctual. Similarly, if you get occasional unwanted thoughts such as 'God does not exist', or an occasional mental image of a corpse in a coffin, or sometimes fear that you are about to make a nonsensical scene in public, there is no cause for concern. Occasional obsessions and/or compulsions are common human experiences. They are a problem if they are frequent and intense, cause distress, and interfere with your life and activities in a significant way.

Some key questions

If you are concerned that you or someone close to you might have an obsessional compulsive problem, these are some questions that are worth asking:

- Do you find yourself constantly avoiding certain things, places, people, or other activities as a result of obsessions and/or compulsions?

- Has your job or other occupation become difficult as a result of obsessions and/or compulsions?

- Do you get very upset by the content or frequency of the obsessions?

- Are you very unhappy about the nature of your compulsive behaviour; for example, is it bizarre or very excessive? Does it leave you open to ridicule?

- Do you find yourself spending a great deal of time engaging in compulsive behaviour or obsessional ruminations?

- Do your attempts to control or resist the obsessions/compulsions take up a lot of energy? Are you often left exhausted by these attempts?

- Are there things that you very much like or need to do, but are prevented from doing because of your obsessions and/or compulsions?

- Is your compulsive behaviour a significant nuisance or hindrance to others?

- Does it cause quarrels and upsets in your family?

- Are your difficulties creating problems in your personal relationships?

If your answer to any of these questions is an emphatic 'yes', then it is possible that your obsessions and/or compulsions merit attention, and you may wish to consider doing something about them.

Concern about a family member

The same considerations apply when a spouse, partner, or any other relative or friend notices compulsive behaviour, excessive reassurance seeking, and so on in a person. It may be that someone spends an excessive amount of time in the bathroom, or gets extremely upset if other people handle his possessions, or insists on keeping his room and possessions arranged in a strictly unchanging way, or expresses an intense fear of contamination or dirt, or engages in extensive avoidance behaviour. Many people with obsessive–compulsive problems attempt to conceal their difficulties from their families and friends, so it may not become clear to them in the early stages that a problem exists.

As mentioned earlier, it is not uncommon for people to feel unsure about whether the problems they (or their children/relatives/friends) are experiencing are manifestations of obsessive–compulsive disorder or some other difficulty. Is it a collection of benign superstitions, or mere eccentricity, or a major mental illness, or a form of autism, or other possibilities? In these circumstances the best step is to seek professional advice.

Finding a therapist

The first step is to go to your own doctor and explain the problem. There is no need to fear that he will think you are peculiar or crazy; and he is likely to refer you to a professional who has specialized knowledge and skills. As explained in the Preface, specialized psychological services are being massively expanded and waiting times are being reduced. Most specialists are clinical psychologists, psychiatrists, or nurse therapists with training in dealing with problems of this kind.

The psychological therapist is likely to be someone with specialized training in cognitive behavioural therapy. As the recently initiated expansion of psychological therapy rolls out, waiting times for treatment should be minimal. In the UK, most therapists work in the National Health Service, but if you prefer to see someone privately, the British Association for Behavioural and Cognitive Therapies will be able to give you advice. General advice on the services of clinical psychologists and psychiatrists is available from their respective professional organizations, the British Psychological Society and the Royal Collage of Psychiatrists. Advice is also obtainable from MIND, which is the National Association for Mental Health, and several other organizations, including First Steps to Freedom, OCD-UK, No Panic, and OCD Action. Details are provided in Appendix 7.

In the USA, the Obsessive–Compulsive Foundation provides information and advice for suffers of obsessive–compulsive disorder and their families and friends. Many have found contact with the Foundation, which is a voluntary and non-profit-making organization, to be extremely useful. Another organization that provides useful information and advice on this disorder is the Anxiety Disorders Association of America.

The therapist's assessment

When you go for your initial assessment, the therapist will try to collect as much relevant information as possible. It may well take more than one interview for him to complete the assessment. The information he is likely to require will include the kind of details discussed in the previous chapters, especially the one on assessment. Your therapist may also give you some questionnaires, checklists, or inventories to complete. He may ask you to carry out short tests. For example, if your problems include a fear of contamination by dirt, he may ask you to touch, with the open palm of your hand, table surfaces, tops of cupboards, door handles, and so on. Alternatively, if you have horrible thoughts and impulses that you might stab someone, the therapist may ask you to hold a knife or a pair of scissors in your hands and to describe to him what thoughts, images, and impulses come to your mind at the time. He may also give you some homework in the form of keeping a diary or record of your problems, as they occur in the next week or two. Cooperate with this even if you think it is a chore. The therapist may also want to see you at home, to see for himself what your problems are and how you cope. Naturally, this will depend on the nature of the problem and on how much time the therapist has at his disposal. Many therapists nowadays, if they can find the time, are likely to include a home visit as a part of the assessment, especially if you are engagng in significant compulsions, such as checking or cleaning, at home.

Planning and implementation of therapy

In planning the treatment programme, your psychological therapist will discuss with you what areas to concentrate on, which targets to set, and how to achieve them. The amount and intensity of the programme will be determined by the severity of the disorder. If the problem is too severe to manage on an out-patient basis, hospitalization for a limited period will be considered as a first step. Hospital treatment will include not only your therapist, but also nurses and other professionals. If your treatment is entirely on an out-patient basis, which is probable, the therapist may conduct, or arrange for, some additional sessions in your home. These domiciliary sessions can be extremely valuable. Irrespective of this, you will be given plenty of advice about what you should and should not do at home.

Do not be surprised if the therapist asks you to continue to keep regular records of what happens at home, since this information is useful in monitoring your progress. He may wish to go over your home records and discuss them in detail at the beginning of each session; the programmes are designed to be self-correcting and the records are utilized for this purpose.

If an ERP programme is undertaken in an out-patient clinic, at least some of your sessions with the therapist are likely to be quite lengthy. Part of each session will be devoted to discussions between you and the therapist about your cognitions—thoughts, images, and impulses. He will want to explore your fears of disaster, the personal significance you attach to the obsessions, your difficulties at home or work, what you really think will happen if you do not carry out your (checking/cleaning) compulsions, how responsible you feel for harm that may happen, and so on.

In summary, your sessions may be lengthy if the major problems are a fear of contamination or dirt, or a fear of being responsible for a disaster. In these instances, the main ingredient usually is ERP. If your main problems are of a different kind, such as repetitive, unwanted, and repugnant thoughts, your treatment sessions will take a different form. If your main problem is obsessional slowness or compulsive hoarding, then much of the therapy may well be home-based.

A word is needed about the involvement of family members. Not surprisingly, family members find themselves in a conflict between providing unconditional sympathy and assistance or refusing to comply with the needs and demands of the patient. Discussions with the therapist are advisable. Families are helped to understand the nature of obsessive–compulsive disorder and the total inability of the patient simply to wish it away or to try harder.

Adjustment problems

As you begin to improve with treatment, you may need to adjust to a new lifestyle, especially if your problems have been long-standing. You will find that you have much free time, and probably not many activities to fill that time with. You may need to develop new ways of using your time, and perhaps new activities. You may wish to revive your impaired social life and resume old friendships and relationships. Your therapist will discuss these matters with you and provide advice and counselling on how to make these adjustments. It is possible that your family members will also have similar problems if their lives had been moulded by your problems.

After therapy

After treatment some of the problems may linger on for a while, but without arousing much discomfort or leading to a strong compulsive urge. You may have minor residual problems, and perhaps continue to be a more anxious person than many others.

Once successfully treated, the chances of a major relapse are low. However, there may be minor lapses. At times of stress (e.g. with problems at work, a death, or a serious illness in the family, and so on) the chances of symptoms reappearing are increased. You can minimize the effects of stress if you use strategies to cope with situations. Relaxation practice is one such strategy (see Appendix 1). If the symptoms of the disorder do reappear, you will notice these signs early on, and can give yourself a few booster sessions using the principles of treatment you are now familiar with. If you need some assistance, a few booster sessions with your therapist are generally sufficient.

It is usual for the therapist to arrange follow-up appointments for you, in order to ascertain how well you are doing, and to give you help and support as needed. If you feel that you are losing control again, contact your therapist, even if there is no follow-up arrangement. It must be reiterated, however, that after a carefully planned therapy programme has been successfully carried out, the chances of the problems re-emerging in full-blown form are limited.

The use of drugs

It is possible that your therapist will consider drugs as part of the treatment, especially in severe cases and for those patients who are notably depressed. As only a medical practitioner can prescribe drugs, if your therapist is not a doctor, he will ask your own doctor or a psychiatrist to consider this. The most likely circumstances for this would be if your mood is depressed and this has either stalled your progress or is making it difficult for you to engage in therapy. In such cases, anti-depressant medication may be prescribed (see Chapter 7). Whatever drug is prescribed, you need to tell the doctor what other medicines you are taking, any allergies that you have, whether you are pregnant, and so on. Make sure you get clear instructions about the dosage, and what foods and drinks (if any) to avoid, and discuss possible side-effects. Commonly prescribed anti-depressant drugs, including clomipramine, have several well-known side-effects (see p. 105).

Two other points are worth bearing in mind with regard to medication. The first is that anti-depressant drugs do not produce results immediately—it may be weeks before any improvement is seen. Secondly, if you are treated just with an anti-depressant drug and no cognitive behavioural treatment, improvements in your obsessive–compulsive symptoms may fade or disappear when you come off the drug.

Brain surgery

It is extremely unlikely that your therapist will recommend brain surgery—unless your problems are very chronic, totally resistant to other forms of therapy, and you are incapacitated by them, this will not even be considered. The NICE report on obsessive–compulsive disorders does not recommend this treatment. If psychosurgery is suggested, you would be well advised to seek a second or even a third opinion. The fullest consultations and discussions are needed.

Self-treatment

Is it possible for someone with obsessive–compulsive disorder to treat himself? Research done in a major London hospital has shown that some patients, especially those with mild problems, can treat themselves. In order to do so, it is necessary first to have an assessment and initial advice from an experienced therapist. Can you do the whole thing yourself, from start to finish? If the problem is mild, and if there are no other complications, this is possible. You need a commitment to the planned treatment, and a systematic approach. If you are seriously depressed, however, then you should not attempt this. Also, if you habitually take a lot of alcohol and drugs, such as benzodiazepines, self-help should not attempted without first consulting your doctor. The nature of the problem is also important. Observable compulsions and unadaptive avoidance behaviour are likely to be more amenable to self-treatment than incessant ruminations or complicated compulsions.

Selecting targets

The first requirement is to select and specify a small number of targets related to your problem. Consider what aspects of the problem you need to improve upon most, then formulate the target specifically. For example, you may decide that one of your targets will be 'to be able to empty the kitchen waste bin into the main dustbin each night' or 'to be able to leave home every morning without checking the gas and electricity more than once'. These are workable targets. More global targets such as 'to get rid of my fear of contamination' or 'to be free of repeated checking and doubting' are less useful, and hard to make use of in treatment programmes. So, be specific in setting targets for yourself.

You should not attempt to tackle too many targets at the same time. It is advisable to begin with just one or two at the most. As therapy progresses, you can add on new targets to your programme as you master the original ones.

Record-keeping

Keeping records is important. They make it easier for you to see your progress, and to identify any difficulties that may arise. For a start, it will be useful just to monitor yourself for a 2-week period, using a form like the one in Figs. 10.1 and 10.2. This will give you a record of the extent of the problem prior to treatment. For recording your actual treatment, use another record sheet—like the specimen form given in Fig. 10.1 (Fig. 10.2 is an illustration of a completed sheet). You will see how all the main details can be recorded on such a form systematically and without too much effort.

Date: Target:[1]

Task[2]	
Time	
Any help[3]	
Discomfort felt[4]	
Urge to ritualize[5]	
Outcome[6]	

1	The particular compulsion treated.
2	Specific task undertaken.
3	Was a co-therapist involved? Who?
4, 5	Rated on a 0–100 scale.
6	Details of what happened.

Fig. 10.1 A specimen record sheet for a treatment session, blank.

Date: Target:[1]

Task[2]	Take kitchen waste bin downstairs and empty into main bin. Clean and reline kitchen bin and place it back in kitchen. Rub handles on clothes and arms. No washing or wiping.
Time	9.15 a.m
Any help[3]	Frances (girlfriend) accompanied me downstairs and back, and encouraged me to rub my hands on my clothes and arms.
Discomfort felt[4]	80 (half-hourly ratings on separate form).
Urge to ritualize[5]	75 (as above).
Outcome[6]	Kept my hands loosely clenched and sat in a corner for some time. Gradually felt better. Had some tea about 10.30. Read the newspaper. On the whole, it went well.

1   The particular compulsion treated.
2   Specific task undertaken.
3   Was a co-therapist involved? Who?
4, 5 Rated on a 0–100 scale.
6   Details of what happened.

Fig. 10.2 An example of a record sheet for a treatment session, completed.

If you are planning to include exposure exercises, it is useful to monitor and record your discomfort and urge to ritualize in graphic form. An easy-to-use format for this is provided in Fig. 10.3 (an example of a completed form is given in Fig. 10.4).

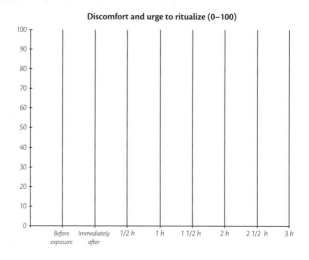

Record level of discomfort with an ∗ and strength of compulsive urge with an O.

Fig. 10.3 A specimen sheet for recording discomfort and urge to engage in compulsive cleaning in an exposure and response-prevention session.

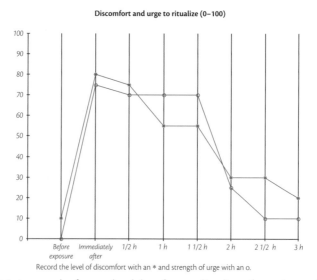

Record the level of discomfort with an ∗ and strength of urge with an o.

Fig. 10.4 An example of a completed sheet for recording discomfort and compulsive urges in an exposure and response-prevention session.

Appraisal of the problem

How you see your problem is important. Having obsessions and compulsions is not particularly unusual or rare, so remind yourself that lots of people have them (see pp. 14–15) and that having them does not mean that you are crazy or that you are going mad. The main problem is the distress and interference they cause in your life and this is what your treatment programme is intended to reduce.

A word of caution

A word of caution is needed about self-treatment. Even if you carry out most of the therapy yourself, it is useful to have your problems assessed by, and receive advice from, a qualified therapist. He will advise you on whether or not a self-therapy programme is suitable, and may agree to see you from time to time to review your progress. It is not advisable to undertake it entirely on your own, unless your problems are relatively mild or you have no suitable therapist available.

Obsessive–compulsive disorders are treatable

It is important to bear in mind that obsessive–compulsive disorder is a treatable condition. Much progress has been made in the last four decades in helping people to overcome these problems. Many, many people with this disorder have benefited from treatment, and significant progress is being made in improving the availability and efficacy of the therapeutic methods. With the provision of correct advice and appropriate treatment, the prospects of improvement are good.

Appendix 1

Learning to relax:
a simple guide

Do your relaxation exercises in a quiet room, at a time when you are not likely to be disturbed. Sit comfortably in a armchair. Make sure that your clothes are not tight. Remove belts, spectacles, and shoes.

Learn to relax by first tensing and then relaxing various muscle groups of the body, one at a time. Keep your eyes closed throughout. At each step, keep the muscles tensed, quite hard, for 6–8 seconds. Concentrate on the muscles, and notice the tension. Then relax the muscles, and keep them relaxed for 45–50 seconds. Again, concentrate on the muscles, and notice how the feelings of relaxation differ from those of tension. You can learn to time yourself quite easily by slowly counting for the first few times. Remember to repeat the tense–relax cycles for each muscle group before you move on to the next. When you tense a group of muscles, take a breath and hold it until you relax the muscles, releasing the breath slowly as you relax.

Given below is the order in which to tense and relax the various muscle groups. For each muscle group, a strategy for making them tense is given. For some, alternative strategies are suggested. Before you actually start the proper relaxation exercises, learn the way in which each muscle group can be effectively tensed. Try out one at a time, and master it. Where alternatives are suggested, decide which one is going to be your regular strategy. Once this is done, you can begin the actual sessions.

1. *Right hand and forearm.* Tense the muscles by making a tight fist; or, try pressing the inner part of the finger tips against the base of the thumb. Relax by slowly opening the hand.

2. *Right biceps.* Tense the muscles by pushing your elbow into the arm of the chair, or by pressing the elbow and the upper arm into the side of the rib cage. Relax by returning to original position.

3. *Left hand and forearm*. As for the right hand and forearm.

4. *Left biceps*. As for right biceps.

   (*Note:* If you are left-handed, do steps 3 and 4 first, followed by steps 1 and 2.)

5. *Forehead*. Tense by raising your eyebrows as high as possible with your eyes still closed. Relax by returning your eyebrows to normal position.

6. *Upper cheeks and nose*. Tense by squinting and screwing up your eyes, and wrinkling the nose. Relax by returning to normal position.

7. *Lower cheeks and jaws*. Tense by clenching your teeth together and pulling back the corners of your mouth. Relax by unclenching the teeth and bringing mouth back to normal.

8. *Neck*. Tense by pulling your chin into your chest, but not quite touching it. Relax by returning to original position.

9. *Shoulders and chest*. Tense by raising and pulling your shoulder blades towards each other. Relax by returning to original position.

10. *Stomach and abdomen*. Tense by pulling in your stomach and abdomen as much as you can. You can also tense these muscles by pushing out your stomach and abdomen. Relax by returning to original state

11. *Right leg*. Tense by straightening the whole leg from the hip, parallel to the floor. Relax by lowering and resting the leg on the floor again.

12. *Right foot*. Tense by pushing your heel into the floor and curling your toes upwards, i.e. towards you. Relax by returning to original position.

13. *Left leg*. As for right leg.

14. *Left foot*. As for right foot.

    (*Note:* If your dominant leg is the left one, do steps 13 and 14 before steps 11 and 12.)

15. *Whole body*. Tense as many of the above muscle groups as you can all at once, making yourself into a 'ball of tension'. You will find that you can tense most of the muscle groups together; in fact, if you use the tension strategies suggested above, there will be only two of these items that you will not be able to do, while doing everything else. One is the raising of the eyebrows, but the eyebrows can be tensed by wrinkling them when

you screw up the eyes. Second is the pushing of your heels into the floor, but, with your legs stretched, you will still be able to curl your toes up towards you.

Remember that each step is to be done twice, including the last 'all body' step. Remember also to take in a breath and hold it when the muscles are kept tense and to release the breath as you relax the muscles.

After the whole sequence is completed, continue to sit in a relaxed state for several minutes. At this point, you may imagine a pleasant scene, such as a peaceful beach or a flower garden. With practice, when you become more skilled in relaxing yourself, you will find that the actual exercises become quite easy. After some weeks of practice, you will be able to relax yourself by simply tensing and relaxing the entire body—i.e. the last step of the sequence given above—without going through the various individual steps. With even more practice, many people acquire the ability to relax very effectively simply by concentrating on making their muscles relaxed without having first to tense them.

If you prefer to do your relaxation exercises lying down on a bed or on the floor, you need only minor changes to the above programme. For each leg, what you will need to do is to raise it from the bed or floor to form an angle of about 30 degrees. Relax by lowering the leg and resting it on the bed or floor.

There is no particular time of the day when relaxation should be practised, but avoid doing it when you are very sleepy, so that you do not sleep while relaxing. Try to do it daily in the early stages, so that you will become good at it.

There are different sequences of muscle groups suggested by different authors for relaxation exercises. There is no particular advantage of one over the others. What is important is to use a sequence that is fairly logical, as the one given here, not a random or haphazard one. You should use the same sequence regularly, so it will be easier to learn and master it.

There are cassette tapes available commercially that give recorded instructions for relaxation training. Using one of these can be useful in the early stages, but it is important to wean yourself gradually away from the cassette, since the aim is to learn to relax without any external aid.

The following are some good cassettes that are commercially available.

Relax and enjoy it, by Robert Sharpe, which is available from Aleph One Ltd, The Old Courthouse, High Street, Bottisham, Cambridge CB5 9BA.

Self-help relaxation, by Jane Madders, available from Relaxation for Living Ltd, 29 Burwood Park Road, Walton-on-Thames, Surrey KT12 5LH.

How to relax, by Rachel Norris and Christine Cuchemann, which comes with *Managing anxiety: a user's manual*, by Helen Kennerley, available from the Psychology Department, Warneford Hospital, Oxford OX3 7JX.

The relaxation tapes (and videos), produced by First Steps to Freedom, 7, Avon Court, School Lane, Kenilworth, Warwickshire CV8 2GX.

Appendix 2

Anti-depressant drugs

Drug	UK brand name	US brand name
Tricyclics		
Amitriptyline	Triptafen, Lentizol	Elavil
Clomipramine	Anafranil	Anafranil
Imipramine	Tofranil	Tofranil, Janimine
Nortriptyline	Allegron	Aventyl, Pamelor
Monoamine oxidase inhibitors		
Isocarboxazid		Marplan
Phenelzine	Nardil	Nardil
Tranylcypromine	Parnate	Parnate
Selective serotonin re-uptake inhibitors		
Citalopram	Cipramil	Celexa
Fluoxetine	Prozac	Prozac
Fluvoxamine	Faverin	Luvox
Paroxetine	Seroxat	Paxil
Sertraline	Lustral	Zoloft

Note This is not a complete list

Appendix 3

The Maudsley Obsessional-Compulsive Inventory (MOCI)

Instructions

Please answer each question by putting a circle around the TRUE or the FALSE following the questions. Work quickly and do not think too long about the exact meaning of the question.

1.	I avoid using public telephones because of possible contamination.	TRUE	FALSE
2.	I frequently get nasty thoughts and have difficulty in getting rid of them.	TRUE	FALSE
3.	I am more concerned than most people about honesty.	TRUE	FALSE
4.	I am often late because I can't seem to get through everything on time.	TRUE	FALSE
5.	I don't worry unduly about contamination if I touch an animal.	TRUE	FALSE
6.	I frequently have to check things (e.g. gas or water taps, doors, and so on) several times.	TRUE	FALSE
7.	I have a very strict conscience.	TRUE	FALSE
8.	I find that almost every day I am upset by unpleasant thoughts that come into my mind against my will.	TRUE	FALSE
9.	I do not worry unduly if I accidentally bump into somebody.	TRUE	FALSE
10.	I usually have serious doubts about the simple everyday things I do.	TRUE	FALSE

11.	Neither of my parents was very strict during my childhood.	TRUE	FALSE
12.	I tend to get behind in my work because I repeat things over and over again.	TRUE	FALSE
13.	I use only an average amount of soap.	TRUE	FALSE
14.	Some numbers are extremely unlucky.	TRUE	FALSE
15.	I do not check letters over and over again before mailing them.	TRUE	FALSE
16.	I do not take a long time to dress in the morning.	TRUE	FALSE
17.	I am not excessively concerned about cleanliness.	TRUE	FALSE
18.	One of my major problems is that I pay too much attention to detail.	TRUE	FALSE
19.	I can use well-kept toilets without any hesitation.	TRUE	FALSE
20.	My major problem is repeated checking.	TRUE	FALSE
21.	I am not unduly concerned about germs and diseases.	TRUE	FALSE
22.	I do not tend to check things more than once.	TRUE	FALSE
23.	I do not stick to a very strict routine when doing ordinary things.	TRUE	FALSE
24.	My hands do not feel dirty after touching money.	TRUE	FALSE
25.	I do not usually count when doing a routine task.	TRUE	FALSE
26.	I take rather a long time to complete my washing in the morning.	TRUE	FALSE
27.	I do not use a great deal of antiseptics.	TRUE	FALSE
28.	I spend a lot of time every day checking things over and over again.	TRUE	FALSE
29.	Hanging and folding my clothes at night does not take up a lot of time.	TRUE	FALSE
30.	Even when I do something very carefully, I often feel that is not quite right.	TRUE	FALSE

Appendix 4

Scoring key for the Maudsley Obsessional-Compulsive Inventory

Instructions

Score 1 when a response matches that of this key and 0 when it does not; maximum scores for the five scales are, therefore: 30, 9, 11, 7, 7.

Question	Total obsessional score	Checking	Washing	Slowness–repetition	Doubting–conscientiousness
Q1	TRUE	•	TRUE	•	•
Q2	TRUE	TRUE	•	FALSE	•
Q3	TRUE	•	•	•	TRUE
Q4	TRUE	•	TRUE	TRUE	•
Q5	FALSE	•	FALSE	•	•
Q6	TRUE	TRUE	•	•	•
Q7	TRUE	•	•	•	TRUE
Q8	TRUE	TRUE	•	FALSE	•
Q9	FALSE		FALSE		
Q10	TRUE				TRUE
Q11	FALSE	•	•	•	FALSE
Q12	TRUE	•	•	•	TRUE
Q13	FALSE	•	FALSE	•	•

(continued)

Question	Total obsessional score	Checking	Washing	Slowness–repetition	Doubting–conscientiousness
Q14	TRUE	TRUE	•	•	•
Q15	FALSE	FALSE	•	•	•
Q16	FALSE	•	•	FALSE	•
Q17	FALSE	•	FALSE	•	•
Q18	TRUE	•	•	•	TRUE
Q19	FALSE	•	FALSE	•	•
Q20	TRUE	TRUE	•	•	•
Q21	FALSE	•	FALSE	•	•
Q22	FALSE	FALSE	•	•	•
Q23	FALSE	•	•	FALSE	•
Q24	FALSE	•	FALSE	•	•
Q25	FALSE	•	•	FALSE	•
Q26	TRUE	TRUE	TRUE	•	•
Q27	FALSE	•	FALSE	•	•
Q28	TRUE	TRUE	•	•	•
Q29	FALSE	•	•	FALSE	•
Q30	TRUE	•	•	•	TRUE

Appendix 5

The symmetry, ordering, and arranging questionnaire

Please circle a number from 0 to 4 to indicate how much you agree with each statement:

	Not at all	Slightly	Moderately	Very	Extremely
1. I feel upset if my furniture or other possessions are not always in exactly the same position.	0	1	2	3	4
2. Other people think I spend too much time ordering and arranging my belongings.	0	1	2	3	4
3. It is essential that I arrange my clothing in a particular and specific way.	0	1	2	3	4
4. I am more at ease when my belongings are 'just right'.	0	1	2	3	4
5. I must keep my papers, receipts, documents, etc. organized according to a specific set of rules.	0	1	2	3	4
6. It is important that my belongings are placed in a symmetrical and evenly distributed way	0	1	2	3	4

(continued)

	Not at all	Slightly	Moderately	Very	Extremely
7. If someone accidentally disturbs my belongings, however slightly, I become bothered or upset.	0	1	2	3	4
8. I feel compelled to arrange my possessions until it feels 'just right'.	0	1	2	3	4
9. When I think that my belongings are out of place, I am uncomfortable or anxious.	0	1	2	3	4
10. When I put my things away, I feel compelled to do it carefully and precisely.	0	1	2	3	4
11. The furniture in my home must be in exactly the 'right' spot.	0	1	2	3	4
12. I feel calm and relaxed only when objects around me are organized and placed correctly.	0	1	2	3	4
13. I feel compelled to arrange cans or boxes of food on my kitchen shelves in a specific way.	0	1	2	3	4
14. When I see that my belongings are out of place, I become anxious until I can arrange them properly.	0	1	2	3	4
15. I feel compelled to arrange objects so that they are balanced and evenly spaced.	0	1	2	3	4
16. I feel calm/at ease only when my surroundings are neat and tidy.	0	1	2	3	4
17. Even when my home is messy, I keep things organized according to a specific set of rules.	0	1	2	3	4
18. Things in my home have a proper and exact place.	0	1	2	3	4

	Not at all	Slightly	Moderately	Very	Extremely
19. I cannot concentrate unless things are in the right place.	0	1	2	3	4
20. I don't like to disturb objects once they are properly arranged.	0	1	2	3	4

The score is the sum of item scores. Scores above 30 are in the high range; low scores fall in the range of 0–10.

Appendix 6

Children's Obsessive–Compulsive Inventory

TO BE COMPLETED BY THE YOUNG PERSON

Date: _____   Age: _____   Sex: Male/Female

Ch-OCI: Part 1

Each of the following questions asks you about things or 'habits' you feel you have to do although you may know that they do not make sense. Sometimes, you may try to stop from doing them but this might not be possible. You might feel worried or angry or frustrated until you have finished what you have to do. An example of a habit like this may be the need to wash your hands over and over again, even though they are not really dirty, or the need to count up to a special number (e.g. 6 or 10) while you do certain things.

Please answer each question by putting a circle around the number that best describes how much you agree with the statement, or how much you think it is true of you. Please answer each item, without spending too much time on any one item. There are no right or wrong answers.

Example:	Not at all	Somewhat	A lot
I feel that I must check and check again that the stove is turned off, even if I don't want to do so.	1	2	3

How much do you agree with each of the following statements?	Not at all	Somewhat	A lot
1. I spend far too much time washing my hands over and over again.	1	2	3
2. I feel I must do ordinary/everyday things exactly the same way, every time I do them.	1	2	3
3. I spend a lot of time every day checking things over and over and over again.	1	2	3
4. I often have trouble finishing things because I need to make absolutely sure that everything is exactly right.	1	2	3
5. I spend far too much time arranging my things in order.	1	2	3
6. I need someone to tell me things are alright over and over again.	1	2	3
7. If I touch something with one hand, I feel I absolutely must touch the same thing with the other hand, in order to make things even and equal.	1	2	3
8. I always count, even when doing ordinary things.	1	2	3
9. If I have a 'bad thought', I always have to make sure that I immediately have a 'good thought' to cancel it out.	1	2	3
10. I am often very late because I keep on repeating the same action, over and over again.	1	2	3

Please try to think about the three <u>most</u> upsetting **habits** that you feel you **have** to do and **can't stop**. For example, feeling that you have to wash your hands far too often, or repeating the same action over and over, or constantly checking that the doors and windows are shut properly.

1)_____

2)_____

3)_____

How much time do you spend doing these habits? Please circle the answer that best describes you.

0	1	2	3	4
None	Less than 1 h a day (occasionally)	1–3 h a day (part of a morning or afternoon)	3–8 h a day (about half the time you're awake)	More than 8 h a day (almost all the time you're awake)

How much do these habits get in the way of school or doing things with friends? Please circle the answer that best describes you.

0	1	2	3	4
Not at all	A little	Somewhat	A lot	Almost always

How would you feel if prevented from carrying out your habits? How upset would you become? Please circle the answer that best describes you.

0	1	2	3	4
Not at all	A little	Somewhat	A lot	Totally

How much do you try to fight the upsetting habits? Please circle the answer that best describes you.

0	1	2	3	4
I always try to resist	I try to resist most of the time	I make some effort to resist	Even though I want to, I don't try to resist	I don't resist at all

How strong is the feeling that you have to carry out the habits? Please circle the answer that best describes you.

0	1	2	3	4
Not strong	Mild pressure to carry out habits	Strong pressure to carry out habits; hard to control	Very strong pressure to carry out habits; very hard to control	Extreme pressure to carry out habits; impossible to control

How much have you been avoiding doing anything, going any place, or being with anyone because of your upsetting habits? Please circle the answer that best describes you.

0	1	2	3	4
Not at all	A little	Somewhat	A lot	Almost always

Ch-OCI: Part 2

In this section, each of the questions asks you about <u>thoughts, ideas, or pictures</u> that keep coming into your mind, even though you do not want them to do so. They may be unpleasant, silly, or embarrassing. For example, some young people have the repeated thought that germs or dirt are harming them or other people, or that something unpleasant may happen to them or someone special to them. **These are thoughts that keep coming back, over and over again, even though you do not want them.**

Please answer each question by putting a circle around the number that best describes how much you agree with the statement, or how much you think it is true of you. Please answer each item, without spending too much time on any one item. There are no right or wrong answers.

Example:	Not at all	Somewhat	A lot
I often have the same upsetting thought about death over and over again.	1	2	3

How much do you agree with each of the following statements?	Not at all	Somewhat	A lot
1. I can't stop thinking upsetting thoughts about an accident.	1	2	3
2. I often have bad thoughts that make me feel like a terrible person.	1	2	3
3. Upsetting thoughts about my family being hurt go round and round in my head and stop me from concentrating.	1	2	3
4. I always have big doubts about whether I've made the right decision, even about stupid little things.	1	2	3
5. I can't stop upsetting thoughts about death from going round in my head, over and over again.	1	2	3
6. I often have mean thoughts about other people that I feel are terrible, over and over again.	1	2	3

How much do you agree with each of the following statements?	Not at all	Somewhat	A lot
7. I often have horrible thoughts about going crazy.	1	2	3
8. I keep on having frightening thoughts that something terrible is going to happen and it will be my fault.	1	2	3
9. I'm very frightened that I will think something (or do something) that will upset God.	1	2	3
10. I'm always worried that my mean thoughts about other people are as wicked as actually doing mean things to them.	1	2	3

Please list the three most severe **thoughts** that you often have **and can't stop thinking about**. For example, thinking about hurting someone, or thinking bad things about God.

1)_____

2)_____

3)_____

How much time do you spend thinking about these things? Please circle the answer that best describes you.

0	1	2	3	4
None	Less than 1 h a day (occasionally)	1–3 h a day (part of a morning or afternoon)	3–8 h a day (about half the time you're awake)	More than 8 h a day (almost all the time you're awake)

How much do these thoughts get in the way of school or doing things with friends? Please circle the answer that best describes you.

0	1	2	3	4
Not at all	A little	Somewhat	A lot	Extreme

How much do these thoughts bother or upset you? Please circle the answer that best describes you.

0	1	2	3	4
Not at all	A little	Somewhat	A lot	Extreme

How hard do you try to stop the thoughts or ignore them? Please circle the answer that best describes you.

0	1	2	3	4
I always try to resist	I try to resist most of the time	I make some effort to resist	Even though I want to, I don't try to resist	I don't resist at all

When you try to fight the thoughts, can you beat them? How much control do you have over the thoughts? Please circle the answer that best describes you.

0	1	2	3	4
Complete control	Much control	Moderate control	Little control	No control

How much have you been avoiding doing anything, going any place, or being with anyone because of your thoughts? Please circle the answer that best describes you.

0	1	2	3	4
Not at all	A little	Somewhat	A lot	Almost always

Scoring of the Ch-OCI

Part 1: Compulsions ('habits')

- Add together the scores of the 10 items (score 1, 2, 3) to get the compulsions symptom total.

- Add together the scores of the first five impairment items (score 0, 1, 2, 3, 4) to get the total score for impairment caused by compulsions. The final item (avoidance) is not included.

Part 2: Obsessions ('thoughts')

● Add together the scores of the 10 items (score 1, 2, 3) to get the obsessions symptom total.

● Add together the scores of the first five impairment items (score 0, 1, 2, 3, 4) to get the total score for impairment caused by obsessions. The final item (avoidance) is not included.

The range of possible scores are:

Compulsions:	symptom score	10–30
	impairment score	0–20
Obsessions:	symptom score	10–30
	impairment score	0–20

Note: The parents' version is the same as the child version, except for obvious wording changes.

*This instrument has been reproduced here with the kind permission of Dr R. Shafran.

Appendix 7

Addresses of useful organizations

UK

British Association for Behavioural and Cognitive Psychotherapies

Globe Centre

PO Box 9

Accrington

BB5 2DG

www.babcp.org.uk

British Psychological Society

St Andrews House

48 Princes Road East

Leicester LE1 7DR

www.bps.org.uk

Royal College of Psychiatrists

17 Belgrave Square

London SW1X 8PG

www.rcpsych.ac.uk

MIND, National Association for Mental Health

22 Harley Street

London W1N 2ED

www.mind.org.uk

OCD Action

Aberdeen Centre

22–24 Highbury Grove

London N5 2EA

www.ocdaction.org.uk

OCD-UK

PO Box 8955

Nottingham

NG10 9AU

www.ocduk.org

No Panic

93 Brands Farm Way

Randlay

Telford TF3 2JQ

www.no-panic.co.uk

First Steps to Freedom

7 Avon Court

School Lane

Kenilworth

Warwickshire CV8 2GX

www.first-steps.org

Triumph Over Phobia (TOP UK)

PO Box 1831

Bath BA2 4YW

www.triumphoverphobia.com

USA

Association for Advancement of Behavior Therapy

15 West 36th Street
New York, NY 10018
www.aabt.org

American Psychiatric Association

1000 Wilson Boulevard
Suite 1825
Arlington, VA 22209-3901
www.psych.org

American Psychological Association

750 First Street, NE
Washington DC 20002-4242
www.apa.org

Obsessive-Compulsive Foundation, Inc.

337 Notch Hill Road
North Branford, CT 06471
www.ocfoundation.org

The Anxiety Disorders Association of America

8730 Georgia Avenue
Suite 600
Silver Spring, MD 20910
www.adaa.org

National Institute of Mental Health (NIMH)

Office of Communications
6001 Executive Boulevard
Room 8184
MSC 9663
Bethesda, MD 20892-9663
www.nimh.nih.gov

Canada

Canadian Psychiatric Association

237 Argyle Avenue
Suite 200
Ottawa
Ontario K2P 1B8
cpa@cpa-apc.org

Canadian Psychological Association

151 Slater Street
Suite 205
Ottawa
Ontario K1P 5H3

Canadian Mental Health Association

8 King Street East
Suite 810
Toronto
Ontario M5C 1B5
www.cmha.ca

Anxiety Disorders Association, British Columbia (ADABC)

4438 West 10th Avenue
Suite 119
Vancouver

British Columbia V6R 4R8

www.anxietybc.com

Australia

Australian Psychological Society

PO Box 38

Flinders Lane Post Office

Melbourne

VIC 8009

www.psychsociety.com.au

Royal Australian and New Zealand College of Psychiatrists

309 La Trobe Street

Melbourne

VIC 3000

www.ranzcp.org

Australian Association for Cognitive and Behaviour Therapy

www.aabct.org

Mental Health Association NSW Inc.

ada@mentalhealth.asn.au

CRUFAD (Clinical Research Unit for Anxiety and Depression)

St Vincent's Hospital

299 Forbes Street

Darlington, Sydney

NSW 2010

www.crufad.org

www.crufad.com

Appendix 8

Some useful reading

Technical

There are several technical books that provide authoritative accounts of obsessive-compulsive disorder.

Barlow, D. H. (2002) *Anxiety and its disorders;* revised 2nd edn. Guilford Press, New York.

> This is comprehensive book on the whole range of anxiety disorders, and has a particularly useful chapter on obsessive-compulsive disorder. Fully revised and expanded.

Clark, D. A. (2004) *Cognitive-behavioral therapy for OCD*. Guilford Press, New york.

> A lucid account of psychological treatments for this disorder.

Clark, D. M. and Fairburn, C. G. (ed.) (1997) *The science and practice of cognitive behaviour therapy*. Oxford University Press, Oxford.

> An excellent volume that covers developments in psychological treatment, including the treatment of obsessive–compulsive disorder.

Craske, M. (1999) *Anxiety disorders*. Westview Press, Boulder, Colorado.

> A detailed comprehensive discussion of the whole range of anxiety disorders.

McLean, P. D. and Woody, S. R. (2001) *Anxiety disorders in adults*. Oxford University Press, New York.

> A clear account of the nature and treatment of obsessive–compulsive disorders and other anxiety disorders.

Menzies, R. G. and de Silva, P. (ed.) (2003) *Obsessive–compulsive disorder: theory, research and treatment*. Wiley, Chichester.

> This edited volume gives up-to-date information on all aspects of obsessive–compulsive disorder and its treatment.

Rachman, S. (2002) *The treatment of obsessions*. Oxford University Press, Oxford.

This provides a detailed account of the nature and treatment of obsessions.

Rachman, S. (2005) *Fear of contamination*, Oxford University Press, Oxford.

A detailed description and explanation of a major cause of compulsive washing and cleaning.

Rachman, S. and Hodgson, J. R. (1980) *Obsessions and compulsions*. Prentice-Hall, Englewood Cliffs, New Jersey.

This book provides a discussion of the field of obsessive–compulsive disorder. It describes the nature of obsessions and compulsions, gives an account of the authors' research, and comments on theoretical issues.

Swinson, R. P., Antony, M. M., Rachman, S. and Richter, M. A. (ed.) (1998) *Obsessive–compulsive disorder: theory, research, and treatment*. Guilford Press, New York.

An edited volume with expert chapters on many aspects of the disorder.

Wilhelm, S. and Steketee, G. (2006) *Cognitive therapy for OCD*. New Harbinger Press, Oakland, California.

An authoritative account by experienced clinician-researchers.

For a shorter account see:

de Silva, P. (1994) Obsessions and compulsions: investigations and treatment. In *The handbook of clinical adult psychology*, 2nd edn (ed. S. J. E. Lindsay and G. E. Powell), pp. 51–91. Routledge, London.

An excellent account of cognitive behavioural treatment by a leading contributor is provided in:

Salkovskis, P. and Kirk, J. (1997) Obsessive–compulsive disorder. In *Science and practice of cognitive behaviour therapy* (ed. D. M. Clark and C. G. Fairburn), pp. 179–208. Oxford University Press, Oxford.

The Vancouver Obsessional Compulsive Inventory (VOCI): Published by Thordarson and others, The Vancouver Obsessional Compulsive Inventory, in the journal, *Behaviour Research and Therapy*, **42**, 2004.

Non-technical

Useful and readable accounts, including self-help advice, are provided in numerous books, including the following:

Purdon, C. and Clark, D. A. (2005) *Overcoming obsessive thoughts*. New Harbinger Press, Oakland, California.

A clear and useable self-help text for dealing with obsessions.

Steketee, G. and White, K. (1990) *When once is not enough: help for obsessive compulsives*. New Harbinger, Oakland, California.

A similarly clear and useful self-help book that covers obsessions and compulsions.

For an account of another anxiety disorder and its treatment, in this Series, see:

Rachman, S. and de Silva, P. (2004) *Panic disorder: the facts*, 2nd edn. Oxford University Press, Oxford.

Index

175